Occupational therapy in the prevention and management of falls in adults

Practice guideline

College of Occupational Therapists

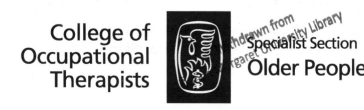

College of
Occupational
Therapists

Specialist Section
Older People

First published in 2015
by the College of Occupational Therapists Ltd
106–114 Borough High Street
London SE1 1LB
www.cot.org.uk

Author: College of Occupational Therapists
Editor: Mandy Sainty
Guideline Development Group: Shelley Crossland, Jo Doubleday, Judi Edmans, Tessa Fiddes, Zoe Foan, Lianne McInally, Catherina Nolan, Kate Robertson
Category: Practice Guideline
Date for Review: 2020

Other enquiries about this document should be addressed to the College of Occupational Therapists Specialist Section-Older People at the above address.

British Library Cataloguing in Publication Data
A catalogue record for this book is available from the British Library.

ISBN 978-1-905944-48-4

Typeset by Servis Filmsetting Ltd, Stockport, Cheshire
Digitally printed on demand in Great Britain by The Lavenham Press, Suffolk

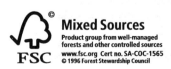

Mixed Sources
Product group from well-managed forests and other controlled sources
www.fsc.org Cert no. SA-COC-1565
© 1996 Forest Stewardship Council

Contents

Foreword by Professor Lindy Clemson   v

Foreword by Dr Jonathan Treml   v

Foreword by Mr Tony Wilde   vi

Key recommendations for implementation   1

Summary of recommendations by category   2

1   Introduction   **4**

1.1   National context: falls statistics   4

1.2   Context of service delivery   5

1.3   Background to clinical condition – falls   7

1.4   Practice requirement for the guideline   9

1.5   Topic identification process   9

2   Objective of the guideline   **10**

3   Guideline scope   **12**

3.1   Clinical question   12

3.2   Target population   12

3.3   Target audience   13

4   Guideline development process   **15**

4.1   Guideline Development Group   15

4.2   Stakeholder involvement   15

4.3   Service user involvement   16

4.4   End user consultation   18

4.5   External peer review   18

4.6   Conflicts of interest   19

4.7   Declaration of funding for the guideline development   19

4.8   College appraisal and ratification process   19

5   Guideline methodology   **20**

5.1   Guideline question   20

5.2   Literature search strategy and outcomes   20

5.3   Criteria for inclusion and exclusion of evidence   22

5.4   Strengths and limitations of body of evidence   22

5.5   Methods used to arrive at recommendations   25

5.6   Limitations and any potential bias of guideline   26

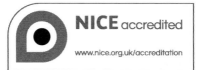

NICE has accredited the process used by the College of Occupational Therapists to produce its practice guidelines. Accreditation is valid for five years from January 2013 and is applicable to guidance produced using the processes described in the *Practice guidelines development manual*, 2nd edition (College of Occupational Therapists 2011). More information on accreditation can be viewed at www.nice.org.uk/accreditation.

Contents

6   The occupational therapy role   **28**
6.1   Identification of people at risk   28
6.2   Assessment of performance and function   29
6.3   Interventions and treatment plans   29
6.4   Self-management strategies   29
6.5   Outcome measures   30
6.6   Staff education and training   30
6.7   Improving health and wellbeing   30
6.8   Multidisciplinary working   31
6.9   Summary   31

7   Guideline recommendations   **32**
7.1   Keeping safe at home: reducing risk of falls   33
7.2   Keeping active: reducing fear of falling   39
7.3   Falls management: making it meaningful   43

8   Service users' perspectives of falls   **51**

9   Implementation of the guideline   **52**
9.1   Dissemination and promotion   52
9.2   Organisational and financial barriers   52
9.3   Implementation resources   54

10   Recommendations for future research   **56**

11   Updating the guideline   **58**

Appendix 1: Guideline Development Group   **59**

Appendix 2: Acknowledgements   **60**

Appendix 3: Conflicts of interest declarations   **62**

Appendix 4: Service user consultation   **63**

Appendix 5: Literature search strategy   **65**

Appendix 6: Evidence-based review tables   **68**

Appendix 7: Glossary and useful abbreviations   **101**

References   **105**

Note: The term 'service user' is used within this document to refer to adults who have fallen, are at risk of falling, or are fearful of falling.

This guideline was developed using the processes defined within the Practice guidelines development manual (College of Occupational Therapists [COT] 2011a).

Readers are referred to the manual to obtain further details of specific stages within the guideline development process.

The manual is available at:
http://www.cot.co.uk/sites/default/files/publications/public/PGD-Manual-2014.pdf

Forewords

Thank you for the opportunity to introduce the practice guideline for occupational therapy in falls prevention. The consequences of falling in older age are a major health and wellness issue for individuals as well as contributing to societal health costs that are accelerating with our increasing older population. On the other hand, the evidence-based interventions we have now can not only significantly reduce the risk of falling but make a difference to the older person's safety, confidence and functional capacity. Occupational therapy in falls prevention is a specialty area. There are unique skills and contributions we can make and I was impressed with the quality and depth of this document. It should be a useful and current tool for implementing falls prevention. The quality is exemplified by the rigour of research into a wide range of service contexts, the careful interpretation of evidence, and relevant examples of implementation issues so important for translation and sustainability. The depth is strengthened by the framing of recommendations across active ageing, enabling and person-centred approaches within three key foci of safety, fear of falling, and managing fall risk. These align with and embrace both fall prevention and occupational therapy philosophy. The profile of those who fall and those who are afraid of falling is different. One does not necessarily lead to the other. Yet both can have dire consequences. I was pleased to see the inclusion of fear of falling and collaborative planning to address risk perceptions, confidence and activity promotion. All the contributors, consultants and reviewers are to be commended. I encourage occupational therapists to engage with this guideline and to use it wisely.

Lindy Clemson
Professor of Occupational Therapy & Ageing
NHMRC CD Research Fellow
Faculty of Health Sciences, The University of Sydney

I would like to congratulate the authors of this guideline for producing an excellent, important and authoritative piece of work. There is no doubt that this guideline will be of great value, not just to occupational therapists but to the wider falls prevention community and consequently to people at risk of falling, or suffering harm from falls. There is much that will be of value to other allied health professionals, nurses and doctors who have an interest in falls prevention. I would hope that this guideline will also be of use in informing health and social care commissioners who have a responsibility for falls prevention.

This document has two particular strengths: firstly, it links a series of key recommendations to a critical appraisal of the evidence base. Secondly, service users are clearly at the centre of this guideline, with the involvement of user groups and the inclusion of illustrative quotes from individuals. This brings the whole thing to life and reminds the reader who this guideline is really for.

Dr Jonathan Treml BA, MBBS, FRCP
Consultant Geriatrician, Queen Elizabeth Hospital Birmingham
Co-Chair, British Geriatrics Society Falls and Bone Health Section

Forewords

I am honoured to be asked to provide a few words for this document. I am a nurse who also has a diagnosis of relapsing remitting multiple sclerosis. One of my more severe relapses left me with a very impaired balance and this in turn led to me falling in excess of ten times a day. The resultant fear of falling was all encompassing and led to me avoiding social activity and being unable to work. This was extremely disabling in all aspects of my daily life; I felt unsafe to perform many routine tasks. At the time I was offered no specialist specific assessment for the prevention of falls.

This guideline offers an excellent framework for occupational therapists to work towards. If I was able to access a service like this during the time I was constantly falling I would have felt far more supported and able to live a productive life. The patient-centred focus of this guideline is particularly impressive and I feel that anyone at risk of or experiencing falls should have access to assessment from a therapist in accordance with this guideline. It is thought provoking for the occupational therapist, and once embedded in practice will lead to better focus on the patients affected by falls.

Tony Wilde
Service User

Key recommendations for implementation

The aim of this practice guideline is to provide specific evidence-based recommendations that describe the most appropriate care or action to be taken by occupational therapists working with adults who have fallen, are at risk of falling or are fearful of falling. The recommendations are intended to be used alongside the therapist's clinical expertise in their assessment of need and implementation of interventions. The practitioner is, therefore, ultimately responsible for the interpretation of this evidence-based guideline in the context of their specific circumstances and service users.

Recommendation statements should not be taken in isolation and must be considered in conjunction with the contextual information provided in this document, together with the details on the strength and quality of the recommendations.

Recommendations are graded based on the Grading of Recommendations Assessment, Development and Evaluation (GRADE) process (Grade Working Group 2004), as described in the *Practice guidelines development manual* (College of Occupational Therapists [COT] 2011a). The strength of the recommendations is identified via a scoring of 1 (strong) or 2 (conditional), and the quality of the supporting evidence via a grading on a scale of A (high) to D (very low). It is strongly advised that readers study Section 5, to understand the guideline methodology, together with the evidence tables in Appendix 6, to be fully aware of the outcome of the literature search and overall available evidence.

The recommendations are based on the best available evidence and so cannot cover all aspects of occupational therapy practice. The three recommendation categories, however, reflect key aspects of occupational therapy in the prevention and management of falls in adults:

i.   Keeping safe at home: reducing risk of falls.

ii.   Keeping active: reducing fear of falling.

iii. Falls management: making it meaningful.

All recommendations were confirmed by the Guideline Development Group (GDG) as being strong (score 1). It should be noted that the recommendations below are not presented in any order of priority or relative importance. The overall quality of evidence grade reflects the robustness or type of research supporting a recommendation, but it does not necessarily reflect the recommendation's significance to occupational therapy practice.

Summary of recommendations by category

Keeping safe at home: reducing risk of falls

It is recommended that:

1.	Service users who have fallen or are at risk of falls should be offered an occupational therapist-led home hazard assessment, including intervention and follow-up, to optimise functional activity and safety. *(Campbell et al 2005 [A]; Clemson et al 2008 [A]; Clemson et al 2004 [A]; Costello and Edelstein 2008 [B]; Gillespie et al 2012 [A]; La Grow et al 2006 [A]; Nikolaus and Bach 2003 [A]; Pighills et al 2011 [A])*	1A
2.	Occupational therapists should offer home safety assessment and modification for older people with a visual impairment. *(Campbell et al 2005 [A]; Clemson et al 2008 [A]; Gillespie et al 2012 [A]; La Grow et al 2006 [A])*	1A
3.	Occupational therapists should consider carrying out a pre- or post-discharge home assessment to reduce the risk of falls following discharge from an inpatient rehabilitation facility, taking into account the service user's falls risk, functional ability and diagnosis. *(Di Monaco et al 2012 [B]; Di Monaco et al 2008 [B]; Johnston et al 2010 [C])*	1B
4.	Occupational therapists should offer service users who are living in the community advice, instruction and information on assistive devices as part of a home hazard assessment. *(Steultjens et al 2004 [B])*	1B

Keeping active: reducing fear of falling

It is recommended that:

5.	Occupational therapists should explore with service users whether fear of falling may be restricting activity, both in and outside the home, and include the promotion of occupational activity within individualised intervention plans. *(Boltz et al 2013 [C]; Kempen et al 2009 [C]; Painter et al 2012 [C]; Wijlhuizen et al 2007 [C])*	1C
6.	Occupational therapists should listen to an individual's subjective views about their falls risk, alongside using objective functionally based outcomes, to determine the influence of fear of falling on the service user's daily life. *(Schepens et al 2012 [B]; Wijlhuizen et al 2007 [C])*	1B
7.	Occupational therapists should seek ways of enabling service users to minimise the risk of falling when performing chosen activities, wherever possible, as this may improve confidence and enable realistic risk taking. *(Wijlhuizen et al 2007 [C]; Zijlstra et al 2007 [B])*	1B
8.	Occupational therapists should facilitate caregivers, family and friends to adopt a positive approach to risk. *(Boltz et al 2013 [C])*	1C

Falls management: making it meaningful

It is recommended that:

9.	Occupational therapists should share knowledge and understanding of falls prevention and management strategies with the service user. This should provide personally relevant information and take account of the service user's individual fall risk factors, lifestyle and preferences. *(Ballinger and Clemson 2006 [C]; de Groot and Fagerström 2011 [C]; Haines et al 2006 [C]; Haines et al 2004 [B]; Stern and Jayasekara 2009 [B])*	1B
10.	Occupational therapists should take into account the service user's perceptions and beliefs regarding their ability, and personal motivation, which may influence participation in falls intervention. *(de Groot and Fagerström 2011 [C]; Gopaul and Connelly 2012 [D]; Nyman 2011 [C])*	1C
11.	Occupational therapists should maximise the extent to which the service user feels in control of the falls intervention. *(Currin et al 2012 [C]; Wilkins et al 2003 [C])*	1C
12.	Occupational therapists should support the engagement of the service user in identifying the positive benefits of falls intervention. *(Ballinger and Clemson 2006 [C]; Nyman 2011 [C])*	1C
13.	Falls prevention and management information should be available in different formats and languages to empower and engage all populations (e.g. web-based support, written information leaflets). *(Hill et al 2009 [B]; Nyman et al 2011 [C])*	1B
14.	Physical and social activity, as a means of reducing an individual's risk of falls and their adverse consequences, should be encouraged and supported through the use of activities meaningful to the individual. *(Rosendahl et al 2008 [B])*	1B
15.	Activities to improve strength and balance should be incorporated into daily activities and occupations that are meaningful to the individual, to improve and encourage longer-term participation in falls prevention interventions. *(Clemson et al 2012 [A]; Clemson et al 2010 [B]; Pritchard et al 2013 [B])*	1A

It is recommended that occupational therapists participate in the national and local audit of falls prevention services, and use the tool available to support this guideline to undertake audit against the above recommendations.

1 Introduction

The prevention and management of falls presents significant challenges for health and social care, magnified by the association of falls with an ageing population and the increase in people living with long-term or chronic conditions.

> **Definition of a fall:**
>
> *Inadvertently coming to rest on the ground or other lower level with or without loss of consciousness and other than as a consequence of sudden onset of paralysis, epileptic seizure, excess alcohol intake, or overwhelming external force* (Close et al 1999, p93).

Falls occur most frequently as a consequence of an interaction between diverse risk factors and situations, some of which can be prevented and others modified. Individuals may not be aware of their risk of falling, and consequently opportunities for prevention of falls are often overlooked, with risk factors becoming evident only after injury, when loss of independence and function may already have occurred (American Geriatrics Society [AGS] and British Geriatrics Society [BGS] 2010). Falls are often attributed by individuals as being an inevitable part of ageing, and a 'trip' or 'slip' may not be identified as a fall. Falls are, therefore, often under-reported and individuals may not be aware that a fall may be a consequence of an underlying condition that could be treated.

The vast majority of statistical data and studies published on falls and falls prevention relate to adults aged over 65 years. Only a limited amount of research has been published examining falls and risk factors for younger adults living with ill health or disability, such as multiple sclerosis (Finlayson et al 2009), intellectual disability (Cox et al 2010) or neurological conditions (Saverino et al 2013).

There is currently no evidence to substantiate whether research reporting on falls prevention and management with older people can be extrapolated to the wider population of adults. It is suggested, nonetheless, that the majority of the recommendations identified within this guideline will be appropriate to service users who fall, are at risk of falling or are fearful of falling, whatever their age or predisposing circumstances.

This practice guideline focuses on the important contribution that occupational therapy makes to the prevention and management of falls in adults.

1.1 National context: falls statistics

The number of people aged 60 years or over in the United Kingdom (UK) is expected to exceed 20 million by 2030, with the number of people aged 65 years or over being projected to rise by 48.7% in the next 20 years to over 16 million. Furthermore, the number of people aged over 85 years in the UK is predicted to double in the next 20 years and nearly treble in the next 30 years (Age UK 2014, Office for National Statistics 2013).

Each year 35% of people aged 65 and over will fall one or more times. Moreover, 45% of those in the 80 years and over age group, who live in the community, fall each year

(Department of Health [DH] 2009, p6). Of those that fall between 10% and 25% will sustain a serious injury (DH 2009).

Adults under 65 years of age may also experience falls. This may be the result of an underlying condition, for example those with acute health problems, or with long-term/chronic conditions such as multiple sclerosis, Parkinson's, early onset dementia and arthritis. Prevalence of long-term/chronic conditions increases with age and the growth in the number of people with long-term conditions impacts further on the health and social care systems across the UK (DH 2013a, Department of Health, Social Services and Public Safety [DHSSPSNI] 2012, Scotland. Scottish Government 2013, Wales Audit Office 2014).

Analysis of a UK national database in 1999 identified that 647,721 people aged 60 years or over attended accident and emergency departments following a fall, and 204,424 people aged 60 years or over were admitted for fall-related injuries (Scuffham et al 2003). Based on current trends, by 2036 there could be as many as 140,000 hospital admissions in the UK each year for hip fractures resulting from falls (Age UK and National Osteoporosis Society 2012, p6). The number of falls and fractures that occur during hospital admission is also a concern, although the number of falls per 1,000 bed-days varies substantially between inpatient service providers (Royal College of Physicians [RCP] 2012). Most people who fall in hospital experience no or low physical harm (such as minor cuts and bruises), but others suffer severe consequences, such as hip fracture, head injury or, on rarer occasions, a fall will be fatal (National Institute for Health and Care Excellence [NICE] 2013a).

The personal consequences of a fall for the individual can be significant. There are also associated financial implications: a hip fracture can result in hospital admission costs of £5,744 per patient and an ambulance callout of £230 (NICE 2013b, p7). The estimated cost of falls to the NHS is £2.3 billion a year (NICE 2013c, p5) and there are also significant costs for social care services. A project exploring a system-wide approach to falls in older people identified that costs were 70% higher in the 12 months following hospital admission for falls, compared with the 12 months before the fall (Tian et al 2013).

The scale and significance of fall-related health and social care issues, exacerbated by pressure on available resources, means that falls prevention and management is 'everyone's concern' (NHS Confederation 2012).

1.2 Context of service delivery

The importance of falls prevention and management services is confirmed by its profile in government, health and social care agendas across the UK. This section refers to some of the core and influential policies and documents, although it does not set out to be all inclusive. Occupational therapists should be familiar with the national and local policies that are relevant to their practice.

Falls prevention and management services traditionally have been targeted at older people. Appropriate falls prevention interventions should be provided for younger adults, although it is recognised that these interventions may be more likely to be delivered within the context of a comprehensive treatment programme for a primary condition.

The *National Service Framework for Older People in England*, launched in 2001, was instrumental in raising the profile of falls prevention, with its aim 'to reduce the number of falls which result in serious injury and ensure effective treatment and rehabilitation for those who have fallen' (DH 2001, p76). A comparable driver is seen in the *National Service Framework for Older People in Wales* (Wales. Welsh Assembly Government 2006). This clearly identifies the need for collaborative working between the NHS, local authorities and other stakeholders to take action to integrate falls and fracture services and reduce the number and impact of falls (Wales. Welsh Assembly Government 2006).

The Department of Health document *Falls and Fractures* identifies four pertinent areas in local service commissioning for falls, falls prevention and fractures. These are improving patient outcomes and efficiency of care after hip fractures; responding to a first fracture and preventing the second; early intervention to restore independence (including falls care pathways); and preventing frailty, promoting bone health and reducing accidents (DH 2009, p2).

The NHS Quality Improvement Scotland (2010, p8) *Up and About* approach is set within the construct of a pathway for the prevention of falls and fragility fractures. The four stages comprise: supporting health improvement and self-management to reduce risk; identifying individuals at high risk of falls/fragility fractures; responding to an individual who has just fallen; and coordinated management including specialist assessment. Allied health profession directors are required to work within NHS Boards in Scotland to support falls leads in community healthcare partnerships to implement integrated falls and fracture care pathways, with a target to reduce fall-related admissions to hospital in people aged 65 years and over by 20% by the end of 2014 (Scotland. Scottish Government 2012, p17).

The *Service Framework for Older People* (DHSSPSNI 2013, pp95–99) outlines the falls agenda for Northern Ireland. This includes a statement that 'older people should be informed of the factors which increase risk of fragility fractures as a result of osteoporosis or reduced bone strength and be able to access interventions to reduce the risk'. One of the quality dimensions in this framework identifies that interventions should be based on evidence of effectiveness that reduces falls by 15–30%.

The Patient Safety Observatory (National Patient Safety Agency [NPSA] 2007) acknowledges that some falls in hospital are difficult to prevent, but note that 'there is much that can be done to reduce the risk of falls and minimise harm, whilst at the same time properly allowing patients freedom and mobilisation during their stay in hospital' (NPSA 2007, p3). There has, as a consequence, been considerable growth in the number of resources available to support a proactive approach to the prevention of falls, the improvement of patient safety, and the reporting of incidents in hospitals (DH 2010, NPSA 2007, Patient Safety First 2009) and in care homes (Social Care and Social Work Improvement Scotland and NHS Scotland 2011).

The British Orthopaedic Association ([BOA] 2007) recognises the integration of falls and bone health services as being of paramount importance. Although there have been some improvements, the National Audit of Falls and Bone Health Services (involving healthcare organisations and care homes in England, Wales and Northern Ireland) highlighted that there is still unacceptable variation in the quality of falls and fracture services (RCP 2010, p5). In 2012 the Falls and Fracture Alliance was launched, bringing together key organisations, including the College of Occupational Therapists, to work in collaboration. The Alliance's challenge is to reduce the rate of hospital admissions for hip fractures and fall-related injuries among older people by 2017 (Age UK and National Osteoporosis Society 2012).

A number of current policy agendas continue to influence the delivery of falls prevention services. Significant among these is the integration of health and social care (DH 2014,

DHSSPSNI 2014, Scotland. Scottish Government 2014, Wales. Welsh Government 2014). Integrated multidisciplinary teams across community, primary care and social care can, for example, target older people at risk of admission, facilitate earlier discharge and promote health and wellbeing. Collaborative integrated working can facilitate coordinated person-centred care and improve the service user experience (DH 2013b).

Evidence-based guidelines are available for the assessment and prevention of falls. The American Geriatrics Society and British Geriatrics Society (2001) published the *Guideline for the prevention of falls in older persons*, which was followed closely by the publication of the NICE clinical guideline for falls (NICE 2004). These guidelines were updated in 2010 and 2013, respectively. The updated NICE falls clinical guideline provides recommendations for all older people aged over 65 years, and people aged 50–64 years admitted to hospital at higher risk of falls due to an underlying condition (NICE 2013c). The prevention of falls and fractures can potentially reduce costs (NICE 2013b), and emerging whole-system data are contributing to the evidence of the financial benefits that may be realised across acute, community and social care services (Tian et al 2013).

1.3 Background to clinical condition – falls

Falls may occur at any age, but the combination of risk factors means that whilst falls are not an inevitable part of ageing, they are more likely to occur with increasing age.

A key stage of any falls pathway for older people is to identify those who may be at risk of falling. Guidance within all four countries of the UK recommends that older people who are in contact with healthcare professionals should be asked about falls experienced in the previous year and, if relevant, the frequency, context and characteristics of those falls (DHSSPSNI 2013, NHS Quality Improvement Scotland 2010, NICE 2013c).

Over 400 risk factors associated with falling have been identified (NHS Centre for Reviews and Dissemination 1996), but these can be divided broadly into intrinsic (person-related), extrinsic (environment-related) and behavioural (activity-related) risk factors (Connell and Wolf 1997, Masud and Morris 2001, Stalenhoef et al 2002) (Table 1.1).

Table 1.1 Fall risk factors (COT 2006)

Intrinsic risk factors	Extrinsic risk factors	Behavioural risk factors
• Previous falls, fractures, stumbles and trips • Impaired balance/gait, restricted mobility • Medical history of Parkinsons, stroke, arthritis, cardiac abnormalities • Fear of falling • Medication (e.g. polypharmacy, psychotropic medication) • Acute illness • Dizziness	• Stairs and steps • Clutter and tripping hazards (e.g. rugs, flexes) • Floor coverings • Poor lighting, glare, shadows • Lack of appropriate adaptations (e.g. grab-rails, stair rails) • Low furniture • No access to telephone or alarm system • Poor heating • Thresholds, doors	• Limited physical activity/exercise • Poor nutrition/fluid intake • Alcohol intake • Carrying, reaching, bending, risk-taking behaviour (e.g. climbing on chairs or ladders) • Footwear • Clothing • Inappropriate use of/refusal to use assistive devices

Table 1.1 (continued)

Intrinsic risk factors	Extrinsic risk factors	Behavioural risk factors
• Postural hypotension • Syncope • Reduced muscle strength • Foot problems • Continence • Cognitive impairment • Impaired vision • Low mood • Pain	• Access to property, bins, garden, uneven ground • Inappropriate walking aids • Pets	

The interpretation of the evidence base for falls risk factors is often confounded due to the variety of study designs employed and heterogeneity of the older population. Studies have, however, identified some people who are at higher risk of falls.

The annual incidence of falls in older people with dementia is around 70–80%, which is approximately twice the incidence of falls in cognitively intact older people (Shaw et al 2003, van Dijk et al 1993). Older people with dementia have a three-fold risk of sustaining a fracture, and among these fractures they have an additional three times greater risk of sustaining a fractured neck of femur (Tinetti et al 1998, van Dijk et al 1993). The highest proportion of hospital admissions for people with dementia occurs where the individual has had a fall, and the second highest occurs for individuals sustaining a hip fracture as a result of a fall (Alzheimer's Society 2009). People with dementia who fall are approximately five times more likely to be institutionalised than those who do not fall (Morris et al 1987).

People with learning disabilities have also been identified as having a higher prevalence of falls and related injuries. There is a relative absence of evidence, but particular risk factors include early-onset age-related degenerative changes, use of psychotropic and antiepileptic medication, behavioural issues and poor risk awareness (Willgoss 2010).

Older people with sight loss are also a high-risk group who are more likely to fall, but vision loss can often be improved by appropriate detection and correction (College of Optometrists 2014). The risk of injury from falls and the rate of hip fractures in this group are nearly two times greater compared with the sighted population (Legood et al 2002, Martin 2013).

Although most falls do not result in serious injury, the negative outcomes of a fall are considerable and can include 'psychological problems (for example, a fear of falling and loss of confidence in being able to move about safely); loss of mobility, leading to social isolation and depression; increase in dependency and disability; hypothermia; pressure-related injury and infection' (NICE 2013c, p26). The costs of rehabilitation and social care are great, with up to 90% of older patients who fracture their neck of femur while in hospital failing to recover their previous level of mobility or independence (Murray et al 2007).

Half the individuals who fall will fall again within 1 year (Close et al 1999). Of particular concern are falls resulting in injuries such as hip fracture and its associated high mortality and morbidity (NICE 2011). It is recognised that recurrent falls have a significant impact on increased rates of hospitalisation, accelerated admission to care homes, lifestyle limitation, quality of life, mobility, independence and self-efficacy (Baker and Harvey 1985, Cummings et al 2000, Gryfe et al 1977, Tinetti 1987).

Fall-related injuries are the leading cause of death among older people. Every 5 hours in the UK, a person dies as a direct result of a fall (DH 2009). Fragility fractures of the spine and hip, in particular, are associated with decreased life expectancy (NICE 2012a). The 'years lost to disability' (YLD) for falls in western Europe rose from around 2.2 million in 1990 to 3.1 million by 2010 (Voss et al 2012).

The importance of a comprehensive multifactorial falls risk assessment to identify the factors pertinent for an individual must be emphasised. NICE recommends that older people should be offered such an assessment if they present for medical attention because of a fall, if they report recurrent falls in the past year, or if they demonstrate abnormalities of gait and/or balance (NICE 2013c).

The most effective intervention to prevent or reduce the number of falls in older people by up to 30% is a multifactorial risk assessment and management programme (Gillespie et al 2012). A multifactorial approach to risk assessment and individual management is the basis of national and international clinical guidelines on the assessment and prevention of falls in older people (AGS and BGS 2010, Australian Commission on Safety and Quality in Healthcare 2009a, Australian Commission on Safety and Quality in Healthcare 2009b, Australian Commission on Safety and Quality in Healthcare 2009c, NICE 2013c). Occupational therapy has an important role within this delivery of effective falls prevention and management across the NICE falls care pathway (NICE 2014).

1.4 Practice requirement for the guideline

Occupational therapy is a key intervention for individuals who have fallen, are at risk of falling or are fearful of falling.

The College of Occupational Therapists Specialist Section Older People (COTSS-Older People) Falls Clinical Forum developed *Falls management* guidance to support occupational therapy staff to implement the national guidance available at the time of its publication (COT 2006). The guidance has been frequently downloaded, used and valued by practitioners, indicating a need for continued information to support evidence-informed best practice.

The 2006 guidance has now been withdrawn and replaced by this practice guideline.

1.5 Topic identification process

The College of Occupational Therapists Specialist Section Older People (COTSS-Older People) identified the prevention and management of falls in adults as the topic for this occupational therapy practice guideline.

NICE has accredited the process used by the College of Occupational Therapists to produce its practice guidelines. Accreditation is valid for 5 years from January 2013 and is applicable to guidance produced using the processes described in the *Practice guidelines development manual* (COT 2011a).

A guideline project proposal was developed by the COTSS-Older People Falls Clinical Forum, in line with the College of Occupational Therapists' accredited guideline development process. This was subsequently approved by the College of Occupational Therapists' Practice Publications Group in March 2013.

2 Objective of the guideline

The guideline objective is:

To provide evidence-based recommendations that inform occupational therapists, working with adults, of their role within the multifactorial assessment and intervention required to prevent and manage falls.

The objective addresses occupational therapy intervention at any point during a service user's journey along the falls care pathway, the stages of which are described, for the purpose of the guideline, as follows (NHS Quality Improvement Scotland 2010, p8):

Stage 1 Supporting health improvement and self-management to reduce the risk of falls and fragility fractures (maintenance phase).

Stage 2 Identifying individuals at high risk of falls and/or fragility fractures.

Stage 3 Responding to an individual who has just fallen and requires immediate assistance.

Stage 4 Coordinated management including specialist assessment.

It is intended that occupational therapists use this guideline to inform their work with service users, with a particular focus on empowering the service user to fully engage and take responsibility for achieving individual goals. It should furthermore inform work with carers and people who support adults who have fallen or are at risk of falls. This may be particularly pertinent when the service user has a cognitive impairment.

The application of this guideline will also inform the delivery of evidence-based services.

This guideline should be used in conjunction with the current versions of the following professional practice documents, of which knowledge and adherence is assumed:

- *Standards of conduct, performance and ethics* (Health and Care Professions Council [HCPC] 2012).

- *Standards of proficiency: occupational therapists* (HCPC 2013).

- *Code of ethics and professional conduct* (COT 2010).

- *Professional standards for occupational therapy practice* (COT 2011b).

- *Occupational therapists' use of standardised outcome measures* (COT 2013a).

- *Occupational therapy for adults undergoing total hip replacement: practice guideline* (COT 2012).

Occupational therapists should also be familiar with their relevant country-specific policy documents and performance measures, and be cognisant of the following guidelines (note the clinical guideline development processes for NICE and the Scottish Intercollegiate Guideline Network (SIGN) have been NICE-accredited):

- *Falls: the assessment and prevention of falls in older people* (NICE 2013c).

- *Quality standard for Falls* (NICE In press).

- *Hip fracture: the management of hip fracture in adults* (NICE 2011).

- *Quality standard for hip fracture* (NICE 2012a).

- *Management of hip fracture in older people* (SIGN 2009).

- *Osteoporosis: assessing the risk of fragility fracture* (NICE 2012b).

- *Management of osteoporosis* (SIGN 2003).

- *Quality care for older people with urgent and emergency care needs* (Banerjee and Conroy 2012).

Occupational therapists must only 'provide services and use techniques for which they are qualified by education, training and/or experience', and within their professional competence (COT 2010, p27). This guideline should be used in conjunction with the therapist's clinical expertise and, as such, the clinician is ultimately responsible for the interpretation of the evidence-based recommendations in the context of their specific circumstances and the service user's individual needs.

3 Guideline scope

3.1 Clinical question

The key question covered by this guideline is:

What evidence is there to support occupational therapy in the prevention and management of falls in adults?

The guideline development group (GDG) members identified, from their knowledge of the evidence base and clinical expertise, key outcomes for falls prevention and management interventions. Outcomes included those pertinent to the individual service user and those of importance to health and social care services:

- Improved identification of people at risk.

- Improved assessment of people at risk.

- Improved intervention to reduce falls risk.

- Reduction in falls risk and rate of falls.

- Maximised functional independence through evidence-based interventions, including positive risk-taking.

- Self-management, incorporating service user and carer/family education and ongoing support and reintegration into community roles.

- Improved understanding of the importance of education and training on the role of occupational therapy in falls prevention and management.

The heterogeneity of the population who fall means that it can be difficult to identify the specific outcomes that will be the most important to an individual service user. A person-centred perspective underpins occupational therapy practice, and intervention must be compatible with the service user's preferred outcomes or, where appropriate, in their best interest (considering lack of capacity and conditions such as dementia).

The guideline scope included searching for evidence in the above areas. Although there were no specific exclusions in terms of interventions, a decision was made that the guideline should focus on interventions that were specifically within the remit of core occupational therapy practice. It is acknowledged that occupational therapists may often undertake, for example, exercise-related interventions, but these are unlikely to be within the competencies of all occupational therapy practitioners.

3.2 Target population

The population to whom this practice guideline applies are adults who have fallen, are at risk of falling or are afraid of falling.

> A **fall** is described as:
>
> *Inadvertently coming to rest on the ground or other lower level with or without loss of consciousness and other than as a consequence of sudden onset of paralysis, epileptic seizure, excess alcohol intake, or overwhelming external force* (Close et al 1999, p93).

To further define the target population:

- Adults are defined as any person aged 18 years and over.
- There are no restrictions or limitations on gender, ethnicity or cultural background.
- There are no exclusions for comorbidities, but each service user should be assessed individually (taking into account relevant comorbidities) when determining appropriate care or action specific to the guideline recommendations.

All populations and subgroups are covered by this guideline, with the exception of people under 18 years of age and people excluded in line with the falls definition, i.e. sudden onset of paralysis, epileptic seizure, excessive intake of alcohol in the absence of any other risk factors, and overwhelming external force.

Falls associated with industrial accidents and sporting accidents were also excluded, as these are usually related to a specific activity and environmental context, involving individuals for whom there are potentially no other significant risk factors for falls.

3.3 Target audience

The principal audience for this practice guideline is occupational therapists who work with adults who have fallen, are at risk of falling or are afraid of falling.

This guideline is therefore applicable to occupational therapy staff delivering services to adults in a wide range of environments across health, social care, voluntary and independent sectors, including hospitals, people's own homes, care homes, day centres and prisons.

This practice guideline will also be relevant to a wider audience, including the following:

- Members of the multidisciplinary team: to provide a greater understanding of the role of the occupational therapist working in falls prevention and management. This will promote closer working between disciplines (including physiotherapists, nursing staff, social workers, support workers, people working in bone health/osteoporosis services, and medically qualified staff), with improved outcomes for service users.
- Social care providers: to support interagency working, facilitating effective discharge and transition back into the community following hospital admission. This will include, where applicable, providers of re-ablement services working to maximise safety and independence and prevent fall-related hospital admissions.
- Managers and commissioners: to provide evidence of the role of occupational therapy with adults who have fallen, are at risk of falling or are afraid of falling, and for use as a reference tool for workforce design and funding models.

- Education providers: as an educational tool, orienting individuals to the occupational therapy role in falls prevention and management (e.g. occupational therapy students, technical instructors, support workers and assistants).

- Private providers and independent sector: a reference point to tailor service provision and staffing to suit this group of service users.

- Equipment providers and trusted assessors: to enhance understanding of the needs of this specific group of service users.

- Service users and their carers: providing information to enable them to be more informed about the occupational therapy process and interventions.

4 Guideline development process

Detailed information on the following steps in the guideline development process can be found in the *Practice guidelines development manual* (COT 2011a).

4.1 Guideline Development Group

Membership of the core GDG comprised seven occupational therapists with expertise in the field of prevention and management of falls, and/or experience of guideline development.

The core group members were all practising therapists or researchers who undertook the guideline development work in their private time. Some members received support from their employers to attend meetings. To facilitate timely progression of the guideline development, much of the liaison and activity was carried out using email correspondence.

Two members of the Research and Development Team and one member of the Professional Practice Team at the College of Occupational Therapists were co-opted as additional critical appraisers, together with five members of the Falls Clinical Forum of the COTSS-Older People.

The Research and Development Manager at the College of Occupational Therapists was co-opted as Editorial Lead.

Given the very specific occupational therapy nature of this practice guideline, it was determined that the core group would be profession-specific, with expertise from other stakeholders and service users obtained outside core group meetings, via consultation with a virtual reference group.

All comments received from stakeholders, service users and end users on the draft scope and draft guideline document were reviewed by the GDG. Where appropriate, revisions were incorporated into the scope form or guideline document before submission for approval to the College of Occupational Therapists' Practice Publications Group. Conflicts of interest declarations were noted and reviewed for any necessary action.

In the interests of openness and transparency, details of the comments submitted as part of the consultation activities are available on request from the College of Occupational Therapists.

4.2 Stakeholder involvement

Stakeholders expected to have an interest in the guideline topic were identified by the core group membership at the preliminary guideline meeting. Specific attention was paid to identifying professional colleagues who may be working as part of the multidisciplinary team and national voluntary organisations that may represent service users.

4.2.1 Scope consultation with stakeholders

All identified stakeholders were approached to comment on an initial draft of the scope, which was provided in the form of a stakeholder information document, together with a comments proforma and conflicts of interest declaration form.

Falls and Fracture Alliance

The Falls and Fracture Alliance, established by Age UK and the National Osteoporosis Society in 2012, was identified as a key collaboration of relevant bodies.

A member of the National Osteoporosis Society agreed to pass the draft scope and draft guideline to members for comment, with replies sent directly to the GDG project lead.

Members of the Falls and Fracture Alliance at the time of the scope consultation included:

Age UK
Arthritis Research UK
Association of Directors of Public Health
British Association for Applied Nutrition
  and Nutritional Therapy
British Geriatrics Society
British Orthopaedic Association
British Society for Rheumatology
Chartered Society of Physiotherapy
College of Occupational Therapists
College of Optometrists

National Care Forum
National Hip Fracture Database
National Osteoporosis Society
Prevention of Falls Network Earth
Royal College of Nursing
Royal College of Physicians
Royal Pharmaceutical Society
Royal Voluntary Service
Social Care Institute for Excellence
Society and College of Radiographers
Society of Chiropodists and Podiatrists

Other organisations and individuals contacted separately:

Alzheimer's Society
British Association of Social Workers
British Dietetic Association
Clinical Commissioning Group Chief Operating Officer
Skills for Care

Comments received were reviewed by the GDG and where these could be endorsed, the scope was amended accordingly.

4.2.2 Draft guideline consultation with stakeholders

The draft guideline document was sent to each of the stakeholders, contacted as part of the scope consultation, for their review and comment. Feedback from other stakeholders (who became aware of the guideline via other circulation channels) was also welcomed.

Responses were received from a number of stakeholders, providing valuable suggestions and advice. All comments were discussed at a meeting of the GDG and taken into account during the revision of the final guideline.

4.3 Service user involvement

4.3.1 Scope consultation with service users

The service user and lay representative groups listed below were consulted on the initial draft of the scope using a stakeholder information document:

- **Rushcliffe 50+ Forum Health Group:** the 50+ Forum is a group of people aged over 50 years who are registered with a general practitioner within the Rushcliffe Clinical

Commissioning Group locality. The Health Group is a subcommittee of the 50+ Forum that focuses on local health issues. Rushcliffe borough is the most southerly borough in the county of Nottinghamshire, bordering Lincolnshire and Leicestershire. The registered population for the clinical commissioning group is 121,000 people, and there are 16 general practices. The Rushcliffe 50+ Forum involves local people who work in partnership with statutory, voluntary and community organisations to develop and improve public services.

- *National Osteoporosis Society members' groups:* two groups of the National Osteoporosis Society expressed interest in involvement in the guideline development, namely the Norwich and Nottingham groups.

The GDG recognised that these groups would not necessarily be representative of all individuals experiencing, or at risk of, falls, in terms of experiences and cultural and ethnic diversity. It was determined, however, that individuals from these identified populations could take on a valuable role in the guideline development process, particularly by providing their perspectives as expert service users and lay representation.

Consultation was by email and post via the Chairs of the Rushcliffe 50+ Forum Health Group and the Norwich group of the National Osteoporosis Society.

The Nottingham group of the National Osteoporosis Society invited the GDG project lead to attend a members' meeting to outline the guideline development process and purpose of the guideline. This was followed up by email and postal contact with members.

Feedback on the scope was positive, and no amendments were suggested.

4.3.2 Draft guideline consultation with service users

Phase 1
Following earlier consultation with the Rushcliffe 50+ Forum Health Group, members who had expressed an interest in continued involvement in the falls guideline development were contacted and invited to discuss the draft recommendations before these were included in the draft guideline to be sent out for stakeholder and service user consultation.

Five people responded to this invitation, and a meeting was arranged to discuss the proposed recommendations and associated outcome statements, scheduled for inclusion in the draft guideline.

Views were sought in particular on the following questions:

- Do you think the explanation of what occupational therapy is and how occupational therapists promote independence is clear enough?
- Do you think the title is right, given that not all falls can be prevented?
- Do you think the recommendations are easy to understand?
- Do you think these recommendations will help people understand how they can reduce their risk of falling?
- Do the outcomes make sense?

The views of the service user and lay representative groups were incorporated into a subsequent draft of the guideline before the wider consultation with stakeholders, service users and end users.

Phase 2
During the main consultation period, further service user engagement took place. Information was sent to the Rushcliffe 50+ Forum and the National Osteoporosis Society member groups inviting comment on the guideline recommendations and outcome statements. The full guideline document was also available for review.

Five service users who had volunteered to review the recommendations and/or guideline also participated in the consultation, three via written or telephone correspondence and two in face-to-face discussions. Younger adults aged 40–60 years were included in this part of the consultation.

Service user and lay representative views and comments on the recommendations established during phases 1 and 2 of the draft guideline consultation are included in Appendix 4.

The meaning of falls to service users, established during the consultation, offers an invaluable insight into the impact of falls on the individual. Some quotes are given in Section 8 or, where applicable, alongside the evidence in Section 7. These statements provide an important user perspective as an adjunct to the published evidence.

4.4 End user consultation

4.4.1 Scope consultation with end users
The target group of end users of the guideline is occupational therapists. Members of the COTSS-Older People were invited to participate in the scope consultation via the College of Occupational Therapists' website where the scope documentation was provided with a request for feedback and comment.

Other Specialist Sections of the College of Occupational Therapists (Trauma and Orthopaedics; HIV, Oncology and Palliative Care; Housing; Work; Rheumatology; Neurological Practice; Mental Health; Independent Practice; and People with Learning Disabilities) were invited to comment.

Comments received were reviewed by the GDG. Where comments could be endorsed, the scope was amended accordingly.

4.4.2 Draft guideline consultation with end users
A one-month consultation period enabled members of COTSS-Older People to comment on a draft of the full guideline.

The consultation was additionally open to any member of the British Association of Occupational Therapists and was promoted via the monthly professional magazine *Occupational Therapy News*. The draft guideline and a consultation feedback and conflicts of interest form were made available to members via the College of Occupational Therapists' website.

All comments were considered for inclusion within the final guideline.

4.5 External peer review

Three independent peer reviewers were identified by the GDG to critically appraise a draft of the full guideline. Reviewers were selected for their clinical and research expertise in the field and/or their guideline development experience or knowledge.

The external peer reviewer form asked for comment on both the presentation and the content of the draft guideline, taking into account factors such as its purpose, robustness and unbiased nature. The detailed views and expert opinions received were discussed by the GDG and used to inform the content of the final guideline.

4.6 Conflicts of interest

All GDG members (core group and co-opted), stakeholders, end users and external peer reviewers were required to declare any pecuniary or non-pecuniary conflicts of interest, in line with the guideline development procedures (COT 2011a). Service users were asked to declare any conflicts of interest.

The nature of the potential or actual conflicts made in the declarations (Appendix 3) was not determined as being a risk to the transparency or impartiality of the guideline development.

4.7 Declaration of funding for the guideline development

This practice guideline has been developed by a group led by a Specialist Section of the College of Occupational Therapists. Specialist Sections are official branches of the College of Occupational Therapists with specialist interests that, through their membership, are able to engage expert practitioners, educators and researchers in the development of guidelines and access the required clinical and research expertise.

As a membership organisation, the major source of funding for the College of Occupational Therapists and its Specialist Sections is obtained from membership. Other sources of income are primarily from advertising and events.

The development and publication of this practice guideline were funded by the College of Occupational Therapists and the COTSS-Older People. The College of Occupational Therapists provided specific resources to cover the meeting venue, travel expenses, literature search, and editorial and publication support. A small research and development grant was awarded by the National Executive Committee of the COTSS-Older People to fund any other costs associated with the development and promotion of the practice guideline.

There were no external sources of funding.

The editorial lead for the guideline was a member of staff at the College of Occupational Therapists. The recommendation statements and guideline content were, however, developed and finalised by the GDG with the involvement of stakeholders, service user representatives, end users and external peer review. The views of the College of Occupational Therapists have therefore not unduly influenced the final recommendations in this guideline.

4.8 College appraisal and ratification process

The guideline proposal, scope and final document were all reviewed and subsequently ratified by the College of Occupational Therapists' Practice Publications Group, in line with the requirements of the *Practice guidelines development manual* (COT 2011a).

The scope was approved by the Practice Publications Group in July 2013, and the final version of this guideline was approved by the Practice Publications Group in August 2014.

5 Guideline methodology

5.1 Guideline question

What evidence is there to support occupational therapy in the prevention and management of falls in adults?

The PICO framework (patient/population/problem, intervention, comparison and outcome) was used to assist in developing the specific practice question further (Richardson et al 1995). PICO describes the specific care group or condition being studied and the nature of the intervention to be investigated. A comparative treatment can be specified where applicable, together with the anticipated outcomes (the desired/undesired or expected results of the intervention) (Table 5.1). This level of specificity is important in developing the question so that it addresses the requirements of the scope (COT 2011a).

Table 5.1 PICO framework

Patient (service user), Population or Problem/circumstance	Adults aged 18 years and over who are at risk of falling, have fallen or are afraid of falling.
Intervention under investigation or action	Occupational therapy.
Comparison (alternative intervention or action)	None.
Outcome desired	• Improved identification of people at risk. • Improved assessment of people at risk. • Improved intervention to reduce falls risk. • Reduction in falls risk and rate of falls. • Maximised functional independence through evidence-based interventions, including positive risk-taking. • Self-management, incorporating service user and carer/family education and ongoing support and reintegration into community roles. • Improved understanding of importance of education and training on role of occupational therapy in falls prevention and management.

5.2 Literature search strategy and outcomes

The literature search was carried out by a College of Occupational Therapists' librarian, an expert in the field of occupational therapy literature, using a search strategy defined following discussion and agreement with the GDG.

The varied clinical and academic experience of the GDG meant there was prior knowledge that the occupational therapy-specific evidence was likely to be limited. On the basis of this, the search covered a wide remit to ensure it was sufficiently robust to locate any relevant articles of which the group may not have been aware.

5.2.1 Key terms

The strategy involved combining concept groups of key words. Five key categories or concepts and their related terms were identified, reflecting in the main the PICO framework categories: falls and related terms; psychological factors; outcomes; interventions; and occupational therapy and related terms. The term 'occupational therap*' was used alone for some searches to enhance specificity (see Appendix 5, Table A1).

Specific exclusions identified were material published before 2003, people aged less than 18 years, and language other than English (due to lack of resources for translation).

5.2.2 Databases

The databases searched reflected the most likely sources of published peer-reviewed occupational therapy and falls prevention and management evidence. Six core databases were searched from 1 January 2003 to the dates the individual searches were carried out (in 2013) as detailed in Table 5.2.

Table 5.2 Database searches

Core databases	
CINAHL	
Medline	
Allied and Complementary Medicine (AMED)	All searches took place during the period 23.09.13.
PsycINFO	
Social Policy and Practice	
Health Management Information Consortium (HMIC)	

Six specialist databases were also searched: OTDBASE; OT Search; OTSeeker; the Cochrane Library of systematic reviews and clinical trials (search date 23.09.13), and the NHS Economic Evaluation Database (NHS EED) and College of Occupational Therapists thesis collection (search date 27.09.13). No date range was set for specialist database searches, with the exception of OTDBASE (01.01.03–23.09.13).

Searches included title, abstract or descriptor fields. The date of each search, search fields and search result numbers are detailed in Appendix 5 (Tables A2 and A3).

Full search histories are available on request from the College of Occupational Therapists.

5.2.3 Search results

The search identified a total of 3,422 results. These were scrutinised for duplicates within both database searches and cross-database search returns by the College of Occupational Therapists' Research and Development Manager. A total of 2,287 duplicates were removed. The unique results list was given to the project lead and GDG members undertaking the screening activity.

5.3 Criteria for inclusion and exclusion of evidence

The resultant 1,135 search findings (title and abstracts) were independently screened by two different members of the GDG (three group members were involved) against an eligibility checklist.

Inclusion criteria were:

- Adults aged 18 years and over.
- Related to falls.
- Occupational therapy or applicable intervention discussed.

Exclusion criteria were:

- Workplace/industry-related falls.
- Sports or leisure activity-related falls.
- Falls related to excessive alcohol intake, sudden onset of paralysis, epileptic seizure or overwhelming external force.
- Grey literature (given the awareness of the availability of a body of peer-reviewed evidence).

Where two screeners disagreed over whether an abstract should be included or excluded for appraisal, the abstracts were reviewed further against the eligibility criteria at a GDG meeting to achieve a consensus.

This process enabled the identification of abstracts that would be potentially relevant to the practice guideline and should therefore be included within the critical appraisal process.

Following the screening, 901 items were further excluded, resulting in a total of 234 items identified for full paper review and critical appraisal. The GDG was alerted to an additional pertinent publication subsequent to the date of the literature search by the library; this met the inclusion criteria and was critically appraised.

A total of 235 articles were critically appraised and their details transferred into evidence tables (see Section 5.4). A total of 33 items of evidence were subsequently used in developing the recommendations (see Section 5.5).

An overview of the literature search outcomes is provided in Figure 5.1.

5.4 Strengths and limitations of body of evidence

Each of the 235 articles identified as potential evidence was critically appraised by two independent reviewers. Appraisals were undertaken by all members of the GDG, with additional support provided by co-opted members. The allocation process ensured that reviewers did not appraise any evidence that they had authored or co-authored. Any discrepancy in grading was reviewed by a third person, and agreement of the final grading was confirmed with the two original reviewers.

The quality of the evidence was assessed initially using forms based on the Critical Appraisal Skills Programme (CASP) checklists (CASP 2013). Assessment took into account factors such as the appropriateness of the study design and recruitment strategy,

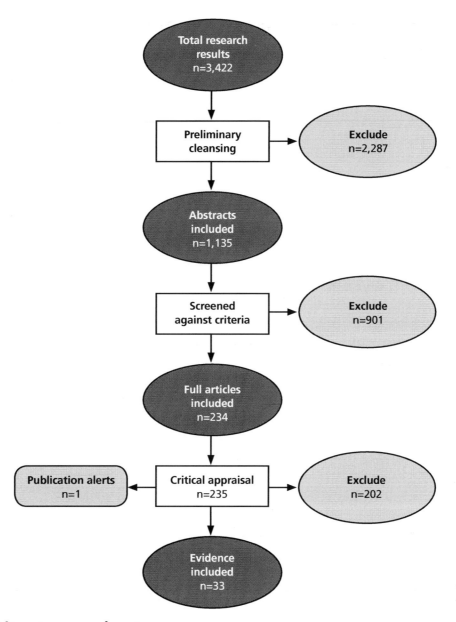

Figure 5.1 Literature search outcomes

procedural rigour in data collection and analysis, confounding factors and potential biases, transferability, precision of results, and the value of the findings.

A quality of evidence grade was then assigned to each individual article using the Grading of Recommendations Assessment, Development and Evaluation (GRADE) approach, as defined within the *Practice guidelines development manual* (COT 2011a). The grading reflects the research design and the confidence in the research findings.

The initial grading was allocated as follows:

• Randomised controlled trial (RCT)/systematic review = High.

• Observational study = Low.

• Any other evidence = Very Low.

Limitations in the design of a study or its implementation may, however, bias the estimates of the treatment effect. If there were serious limitations, then downgrading of the quality of the evidence was considered, as in Table 5.3.

Table 5.3 Grading evidence up or down (after GRADE Working Group 2004)

Decrease* grade if *Each quality criterion can reduce the quality by one or, if very serious, two levels.	• Serious or very serious limitation to study quality • Important inconsistencies in results • Some or major uncertainty about directness of the evidence • Imprecise or sparse data (relatively few participants or events) • High probability of reporting bias
Increase grade if	• Magnitude of treatment effect is very large and consistent • Evidence of large dose–response relationship • All plausible confounders/biases would have decreased magnitude of an apparent treatment effect *Only studies with no major threats to validity should be upgraded*

A decision to increase or decrease the initial grade of the evidence was recorded and justified on the critical appraisal forms. A moderate category became relevant only if there was a suggested change in the initial grading of an article due to up- or downgrading. Evidence was ultimately graded in one of four categories, as detailed in Table 5.4. If there was no reason to up- or downgrade the evidence, then the original grading remained.

Table 5.4 GRADE quality of evidence grading (after GRADE Working Group 2004)

Quality of evidence	Grading	Characteristics	Confidence
High	A	Based on consistent results from well-performed randomised controlled trials, or overwhelming evidence of an alternative source, e.g. well-executed observational studies with strong effects.	True effect lies close to that of the estimate of the effect. Further research very unlikely to change confidence in the estimate of the effect.
Moderate	B	Based on randomised controlled trials where there are serious flaws in conduct, inconsistency, indirectness, imprecise estimates, reporting bias or some other combination of these limitations, or from other study designs with special strengths.	True effect likely to be close to the estimate of the effect, but there could be a substantial difference. Further research is likely to have an important impact on confidence in the estimate of the effect and may change the estimate.
Low	C	Based on observational evidence, or from controlled trials with several very serious limitations.	True effect may be substantially different from the estimate of the effect. Further research very likely to have an important impact on confidence in the estimate of the effect and is likely to change the estimate.
Very low	D	Based on case studies or expert opinion.	Any estimate of effect is very uncertain and may be far from the true effect.

Once the methodological quality of each piece of evidence was assessed, details for each item of evidence were collated into an evidence-based review table (see Appendix 6).

5.5 Methods used to arrive at recommendations

The evidence tables were used by the GDG to synthesise the evidence available and as the basis to evaluate and judge the potential contribution of each item of evidence to the development of the guideline recommendations.

The identified outcomes (see Section 3.1) were used as the starting point in conjunction with themes identified from the appraised evidence. Where evidence was identified to support an outcome or theme, this was reviewed. Each individual group member contributed their expert views to the discussion to develop recommendation options.

Where a number of items of evidence supported an identified outcome and subsequent recommendation, an overall quality of evidence GRADE rating was determined. This overall rating was established as follows:

- Where the evidence outcomes pointed in different directions towards both benefit and harm, the lowest quality grade of evidence determined the overall quality of evidence.

- Where the outcomes pointed in the same direction towards either benefit or harm, the highest grade of quality of evidence was appropriate to recommend an intervention and determined the overall quality of evidence.

- Where the balance of benefits and harm was uncertain, the lowest grade of quality of evidence was assigned.

Strength of recommendation was the second element of the GRADE system applied using the categories 'strong' or 'conditional' to reflect the strength (see Table 5.5).

Table 5.5 Strength of grade (after Guyatt et al 2008)

Strength	Grade	Benefits and risks	Implications
Strong	1 'It is recommended . . .'	Benefits appear to outweigh the risks (or vice versa) for the majority of the target group.	Most service users would want or **should** receive this course of intervention or action.
Conditional	2 'It is suggested . . .'	Risks and benefits are more closely balanced, or there is more uncertainty in likely service user values and preferences.	The majority of service users would want this intervention but not all, and therefore they should be supported to arrive at a decision for intervention consistent with the benefits and their values and preferences.

The development of the recommendations, including assignment of the overall quality and strength grading, was a consensus decision obtained at the GDG meeting and by subsequent email correspondence as required for any revisions. There were no recommendations that were not agreed by all members, and so no formal voting system or use of the nominal group technique was required. A total of 33 items of evidence were used to develop the recommendations.

A recommendation decision form was completed for each recommendation developed. This form recorded key information about the evidence used to form the basis of that recommendation, the overall allocation of the quality of evidence, and the strength of the recommendation. The form also facilitated discussion and recording of any specific or associated risks and benefits, and this was reflected in the final strength of recommendation. Any judgement by the GDG was documented as part of this decision-making process. (The forms are available on request from the College of Occupational Therapists.)

5.6 Limitations and any potential bias of guideline

Evidence included in the development of the guideline recommendations was sourced from published peer-reviewed journal articles. Relevant policy documents and grey literature have been referenced within the contextual information, where applicable.

The outcome of the literature search, appraisal and synthesis of the evidence resulted in 33 papers being used to support the guideline recommendations. The guideline group downgraded 11 of these studies, initially graded A, due to limitations identified from the appraisal and a resultant lack of confidence in the estimate of the research effect. These decisions and comments on individual studies are noted in the evidence tables in Appendix 6.

Over half of the evidence used was derived from studies of high or moderate quality:

- Grade A = 24.3% (n=8)
- Grade B = 33.3% (n=11)
- Grade C = 39.4% (n=13)
- Grade D = 3.0% (n=1)

The literature search identified a body of primary occupational therapy research, predominantly within the area of home hazards and environmental assessment and intervention. The evidence did, however, have a number of limitations; this was particularly evident with respect to the lack of diversity of the participants. Most studies also had a bias towards female participants being recruited.

The inclusion criteria of most of the studies focused on older people (aged over 60, 65 or 70 years), community settings, and those without impaired cognition. Most studies excluded participants with cognitive deficits, despite the fact that cognitive impairment is an important risk factor for falls. The lack of research in the area of fall-prevention interventions for older people with mental health conditions, and the inconclusive evidence that does exist, has been highlighted within systematic reviews (Bunn et al 2014, Winter et al 2013).

Substantiation of the applicability of the recommendations to the wider population of adults who fall or are at risk of falling cannot currently be evidenced. It is suggested, however, that the majority of the recommendations will be appropriate to service users who fall, are at risk of falling or are fearful of falling, whatever their predisposing circumstances. Implementation of the recommendations should, nonetheless, take place in the context of the occupational therapist's clinical reasoning and the individual needs of the service user.

It is important to highlight that this guideline is based on the best available evidence, and subsequently the recommendations cannot explicitly address all clinical, health and social care areas or outcomes identified within the scope. The guideline does not therefore reflect the full range of interventions used by occupational therapists in the prevention and management of falls.

The role of the College of Occupational Therapists and the COTSS-Older People in the development, authoring and funding of this practice guideline is fully acknowledged (see Section 4.7). Involvement is inherent because of the organisational structure of the professional body and its relationship with members of the British Association of Occupational Therapists.

The potential for any bias in development and authoring was minimised through the rigorous nature of the guideline development process. This was achieved through the systematic methodology adopted, the contributions of stakeholders and service users, and the valued opinions of the external peer reviewers and occupational therapy end users.

6 The occupational therapy role

Occupational therapy intervention with adults who have fallen, are at risk of falling or are fearful of falling occurs in a wide range of settings in health, social care, voluntary and independent sectors, including hospitals, people's own homes, care homes, day centres and prisons.

The person-centred and holistic philosophy of occupational therapy underpins the recommendations within this guideline. The purpose of occupational therapy is to enable people to fulfil, or to work towards fulfilling, their needs and wishes in their lives. Occupational therapy provides practical support to enable people to overcome any barriers that prevent them from doing the activities (occupations) that matter to them. This helps to increase people's independence and maintain their dignity and satisfaction in all aspects of life. 'Occupation' refers to practical and meaningful activities that allow people to achieve their wishes and meet their needs. This could be essential day-to-day tasks such as getting dressed, work-related activities, or leisure activities and hobbies.

Clinical reasoning must take account of individual preferences and needs, including the complexities of treating people with multiple pathologies and people with cognitive or emotional disorders, dementia and learning disabilities.

Occupational therapists consider the person, their environment and their occupation (Law et al 1996). These three domains have an alignment with the risk factor categories for falls: intrinsic (person), extrinsic (environment) and behavioural (occupation). Embracing the three means that occupational therapy falls prevention and management intervention maximises the potential to impact positively on an individual's ability to carry out daily activities ('occupational performance').

The occupational therapy role in falls prevention and management may include, but is not necessarily limited to, the key areas described in the sections below:

6.1 Identification of people at risk

Identifying people at risk is in line with NICE Clinical Guideline 161, which states that 'older people in contact with healthcare professionals should be asked routinely whether they have fallen in the past year and asked about the frequency, context and characteristics of the fall/s' (NICE 2013c, p11).

Falls, osteoporosis and osteoporotic fractures are inextricably linked, and occupational therapists should therefore be aware of higher-risk groups, and the importance of diet, medication and (bone-loading) physical activity, applying, as appropriate, any associated clinical guidance (NICE 2012b, SIGN 2003).

NICE identifies 'older people' as people aged 65 years and over, but in the case of hospital admissions also includes people aged 50–64 years who are deemed at risk of falling due to an underlying condition. Occupational therapists work with adults of all ages who may be at risk or fearful of falling in a variety of settings, such as people living with Parkinson's who are at increased risk of falling due to postural instability, impaired balance, reduced saving reactions, visuospatial disturbances and difficulties with tasking (Aragon and Kings 2010, p34); people who have had lower limb amputations (COT 2011c); and people undergoing total hip replacement (COT 2012). The occupational therapist, therefore, needs to be able to identify an individual's risk factors for falls, including those factors that can and cannot be modified.

6.2 Assessment of performance and function

Occupational therapists contribute to a number of the elements of a multifactorial assessment, notably with respect to the 'assessment of perceived functional ability and fear relating to falling', and 'assessment of home hazards' (NICE 2013c, p13).

Assessment includes an individual's ability to perform activities of daily living that they need or wish to perform independently and safely (e.g. getting dressed, cooking a meal, walking outside), roles (e.g. returning to work, caring for another person), social and psychological considerations, cognition, fear and confidence, and mental capacity.

6.3 Interventions and treatment plans

Interventions include positive risk-taking in activity, maximising functional performance, improving self-confidence and social engagement. Environmental advice and modification to reduce home hazards, education and practice in safe moving and handling, with provision of equipment as required, are also appropriate. All interventions should promote independence and personal safety. Reablement, where indicated, will involve working with support workers to resume activities of daily living and occupational roles (Social Care Institute for Excellence [SCIE] and COT 2011).

Occupational therapy intervention for falls may be in the context of condition management strategies. A pilot study in Australia examined the potential for the inclusion of occupational therapy and physiotherapy services within chronic disease management plans in the primary care setting; results demonstrated encouraging outcomes for reducing falls risk (Mackenzie and Clemson 2014).

6.4 Self-management strategies

Falls prevention education and information for service users should be congruent with the NICE clinical guideline (NICE 2013c). Information should include actions or behaviours that the service user can use to prevent further falls; how to stay motivated if referred for falls prevention intervention that includes exercise or strength and balancing components; the preventable nature of some falls; the physical and psychological benefits of modifying falls risk; and where to seek further advice. Where a service user requires assistance to implement self-management strategies (e.g. as a consequence of a poor level of risk awareness due to cognitive impairment or learning disability), there is a role for occupational therapists in supporting the person's carers and family. Occupational therapists have a key role in signposting to falls prevention advice and support available locally and nationally.

Contingency planning for the management of future falls that may occur should be explored. This may include advice and practice, where appropriate, on how to summon help and how to avoid the consequences of a 'long lie'. Occupational therapists should help the service user identify behaviours that may increase the risk of falls and assist with behaviour change to reduce those risks.

Telecare (technology such as a pendant alarm to summon assistance, or remote monitoring via items such as a falls detector) is an option which may be explored in the context of self-management. The evidence remains mixed with regard to telecare outcomes and cost-effectiveness (Henderson et al 2013, Steventon et al 2013). Qualitative studies have identified that when tailored sensitively to the needs of the individual, telecare has the potential to increase confidence and reduce fear of falling (Horton 2008, Stewart and McKinstry 2012). The use of technology is likely to be influenced by intrinsic factors associated with the individual's attitude, choice, control, independence and perceived need for safety measures (Hawley-Hague et al 2014).

6.5 Outcome measures

Occupational therapists working in partnership with people who fall, are at risk of falling or are fearful of falling should evaluate the effectiveness of their intervention. This means ensuring that appropriate standardised assessment tools are used as a baseline from which change can be measured (COT 2014), seeking the views of individuals and carers regarding the effectiveness of the intervention, and documenting the process and results of assessments and interventions. Records and outcome measures should be used to ensure progress is made towards the agreed goals and objectives (COT 2006, COT 2013a).

The COTSS-Older People Falls Clinical Forum provides an opportunity for occupational therapists to review and discuss current evidence and practice in relation to standardised assessments for falls.

6.6 Staff education and training

Occupational therapists provide a crucial contribution to the education and training of other staff working in falls prevention and support the delivery of the NICE recommendation that 'all healthcare professionals dealing with patients known to be at risk of falling should develop and maintain basic professional competence in falls assessment and prevention' (NICE 2013c, p16). In addition to traditional healthcare settings, the occupational therapist has an important role in working with and training staff in care homes (COT 2013b) and care workers delivering home care services and reablement (SCIE and COT 2011).

6.7 Improving health and wellbeing

Improving health, wellbeing and independence, including reducing falls, is a public health priority (DH and Public Health England 2014). It is important, therefore, to note that it is being increasingly recognised that allied health professionals 'have the potential to add to virtually every public health priority' (Hindle 2014). Public health guidance also identifies that occupational therapists have a valuable contribution in promoting mental wellbeing through physical activity interventions (NICE 2008). The public health guidance complements and supports the falls guideline (NICE 2013c), and occupational therapists should therefore explore and support opportunities for service users to participate in appropriate physical activity. Occupational therapists should also take into account potential health inequalities and any social determinants of health, which may be appropriate to the provision of services. In falls prevention and management, this can be addressed specifically through maximising individual capacity and control over life and strengthening the role and impact of ill health prevention (Marmot 2010, p15).

6.8 Multidisciplinary working

The multifactorial nature of falls prevention and management strategies means that working as an effective team member is vital. It is recognised that as part of a multidisciplinary team, there may be some key areas of assessment and intervention that overlap with the role of other health and social care personnel. Where an occupational therapist is unable to provide the required intervention, the service user should be referred to an appropriate service to meet his or her needs (COT 2006, p10).

Occupational therapy staff must work alongside other professionals in accordance with local service arrangements to ensure the needs of the service user are met. Good communication across the primary and secondary care interface, and between health, social care and the independent and voluntary sectors, is imperative.

6.9 Summary

Health and social care services continue to move forward at pace. The move towards integrated working, generic roles and multidisciplinary teams means it is important that the roles of different professions and team members are clearly understood. This is vital to ensure that service users can benefit from the range of expertise available to them and that specialist skills are used effectively in falls prevention and management services.

This guideline provides evidence-based recommendations for occupational therapists delivering services. It also sets out to increase understanding about the role of occupational therapy in the prevention and management of falls. In the context of the impact of falls and fractures on the individual, and the resulting treatment costs across the whole health and social care system (NICE 2013b, Tian et al 2013), the inclusion of occupational therapists as core members of falls prevention and management services should be considered by managers and commissioners as cost-efficient.

7 Guideline recommendations

The recommendations developed by the GDG are underpinned by the available evidence. Synthesis of that evidence resulted in the emergence of three core themes and associated outcomes applicable to occupational therapy interventions:

- Keeping safe at home: reducing risk of falls.

- Keeping active: reducing fear of falling.

- Falls management: making it meaningful.

The three themes cut across the outcomes identified within the guideline question (see Section 5.1 and Table 5.1). Although the recommendation statements have been set out within three categories, it is essential to recognise that there are overlaps. In many cases there is a strong interface across them all. Recommendations should not be considered in isolation but in the wider context, taking into account the body of evidence.

Where applicable, qualitative service user feedback has been used to provide a user perspective as an adjunct to the published evidence.

The strength of the recommendations is identified via a scoring of 1 (strong) or 2 (conditional), and the quality of the supporting evidence via a grading on a scale of A (high) to D (very low). A recommendation grading takes into account the consistency in the direction of the outcomes from the individual items of evidence used to support that recommendation.

All recommendations were agreed by the GDG as being strong, that is, most service users would want to, or *should* receive, the course of intervention or action stated.

Additional details on individual studies (e.g. study design, methodological limitations, recruitment numbers, statistical significance) can be accessed in the evidence-based review tables in Appendix 6.

Outcomes sought, risks, generalisability and social determinants of health associated with each category of recommendations are outlined in Sections 7.1.3, 7.2.3 and 7.3.3. Financial and organisational barriers are discussed in Section 9.2.

This guideline focuses specifically on occupational therapy, as defined in the scope, and therefore does not set out to compare occupational therapy with other interventions. This is in line with the PICO framework (Richardson et al 1995), which for this guideline, did not specify a comparative intervention (see Section 5.1). Alternative management options are therefore not explicitly reviewed or discussed. Occupational therapists should, however, be aware of other interventions that may be available from other members of the multidisciplinary team as part of multifactorial intervention, such as strength and balance training, exercise, vision assessment and referral, and medication review (NICE 2013c, pp14–15).

Recommendations are based on synthesis of the best available evidence. It should therefore be noted that the guideline is not able to be fully reflective of the role of occupational therapy (see Section 6) in the prevention and management of falls in adults.

7.1 Keeping safe at home: reducing risk of falls

7.1.1 Introduction

The NICE (2013c) and AGS and BGS (2010) guidelines for falls recommend that a multifactorial falls risk assessment should be offered to older people who present for medical attention because of a fall, or recurrent falls during the previous 12 months. Home hazard assessment and intervention is identified as one component of this multifactorial approach.

Occupational therapy should be an integral part of a multifactorial falls prevention programme; occupational therapists have significant skills and expertise in the delivery of home hazards assessment and safety interventions. Environmental assessment must be conceived as greater than a 'checklist' determination of home hazards. It is essential that the assessment explores how the actual use of the environment influences the individual's risk of falling. The willingness of service users to accept help with removing or modifying home hazards may be influenced by a number of factors; one large cross-sectional study in the UK identified that these included older age, recent falls and lower economic status (Yardley et al 2008). Fundamental to home hazard assessment and subsequent interventions and follow-up is, therefore, the issue of motivation and engagement (see Section 7.3).

Person-centred and occupation-focused interventions are provided by occupational therapists, in which 'the physical and psychological benefits of maintaining independence are weighed against potential physical damage if an injury occurs as a result of a fall' (Chase et al 2012, p288). The occupational therapist acknowledges the dynamic relationship between the individual and his or her environment; home hazards and behaviour are modifiable whereas some medical falls risks are not.

> *When helping to remove and reduce someone's falls risk, occupational therapists take a broad holistic view and work together with the individual client to consider factors within each of these domains [person, environment and occupation] and how they interact.* (Ballinger and Brooks 2013, p2)

Provision of occupational therapy within this multifactorial context includes the concurrent potential for a positive impact on activities of daily living, notably mobility and bathing (Chase et al 2012, Gitlin et al 2006, Tolley and Atwall 2003). It is acknowledged, however, that by providing a combination of interventions, determining which part of a programme contributes directly to improvements for the service user can be complex.

The evidence and recommendations set out in this section are considered within the framework of the NICE recommendations for home hazard and safety intervention (NICE 2013c, p15):

> *Older people who have received treatment in hospital following a fall should be offered a home hazard assessment and safety intervention/modifications by a suitably trained healthcare professional. Normally this should be part of discharge planning and be carried out within a timescale agreed by the patient or carer, and appropriate members of the health care team.* (Recommendation 1.1.6.1)

> *Home hazard assessment is shown to be effective only in conjunction with follow up and intervention, not in isolation.* (Recommendation 1.1.6.2)

The gap in access to home hazard assessment and intervention has, however, been highlighted in the National Audit of Falls and Bone Health in Older People (RCP 2010). The audit identified that only '65% of patients with hip fracture and 19% of patients with non-hip fracture' received home hazard assessment by an occupational therapist. Of those, less than half took place in the service user's home environment (RCP 2010 p7).

The evidence reviewed has been considered with specific regard to the role of the occupational therapist within the delivery of the NICE recommendations.

7.1.2 Evidence

An Australian randomised controlled trial set out to test whether a multifaceted community-based programme (Stepping On) facilitated by an occupational therapist was effective in reducing falls in people aged 70 years or over, living at home and at risk of falls (**Clemson et al 2004**). Participants had experienced a fall in the previous 12 months or had concerns about falling.

The Stepping On programme principles were to 'improve fall self-efficacy, encourage behavioural change, and reduce falls'. The programme included sessions about balance and strength exercises and moving about safely; home hazards (identifying and problem solving); community safety and footwear; vision; vitamin D and hip protectors; management of medication and mobility techniques (including in the community). The programme incorporated a number of learning strategies, such as 'raising awareness; targeting those behaviours that had the most effect on reducing risk and reinforcing their application to the individual's home and community setting; specific techniques such as storytelling, mastery experiences, and the group process as a learning environment'.

The intervention group (n=157) attended two-hour group sessions, facilitated by an occupational therapist, on a weekly basis for seven weeks. There was an average of 12 participants per group. A subsequent follow-up occupational therapy home visit was conducted; the environment assessment included recommendations for removing or modifying home fall hazards such as removal of clutter, increased lighting levels, application of non-slip tape to step edges and fixing pathways. Seventy per cent of participants in the programme actioned at least 50% of the home visit recommendations. The control group received up to two social visits when falls or falls prevention were not discussed (n=153). A 31% reduction in falls was experienced within the intervention group; secondary analysis identified the programme was particularly effective for men.

A more recent UK study aimed to assess the effectiveness of environmental falls prevention for people aged 70 years and over, living in the community and with a history of one or more falls over the previous year (**Pighills et al 2011**). The randomised controlled trial involved three arms; participants were randomised to either an environmental assessment led by an occupational therapist (n=87), an environmental assessment led by a trained assessor (n=73) or usual care in the control group (n=78). The Westmead Home Safety Assessment was used to assess the participants in their home environment and identified personal risk from both environmental and behavioural perspectives. Fall hazards were discussed and recommendations agreed. Follow-up took place at 3, 6 and 12 months via questionnaire. There was no significant effect from the intervention on fear of falling. The study results determined, however, that the group receiving the assessment led by the occupational therapist had significantly fewer falls than the control group 12 months after the assessment. Within the trained assessor group, there was no significant effect on falls. This important pilot study identified that the professional background of the person who delivered the environmental assessment and home modification intervention influenced the effectiveness of the outcome. Occupational therapists were more effective than trained assessors in identifying the need for modification, and in their influence on adherence to recommendations and the reduction of falls in high-risk individuals.

Nikolaus and Bach (2003) conducted a randomised controlled trial that examined the effectiveness of a home assessment and intervention programme in reducing falls among older people (mean age 81 years) living in Germany. The intervention group consisted of 181 participants. During their hospital stays, the home interventions team (an occupational therapist, together with a nurse or physiotherapist) carried out a home visit to evaluate the person's home and prescribe appropriate equipment. After discharge, at least one further home visit was carried out. The control group (n=179) received usual care but no home visits. Follow-up at one year identified that the intervention group had 31% fewer falls than the control group, with the intervention being most effective for people who reported two or more falls. The intervention for this subgroup resulted in a significant reduction in the rate of falls and proportion of frequent fallers compared with the control group.

> *"More home assessments are needed."*
>
> Volunteer at the Involvement Centre in Nottingham

The **Campbell et al (2005)** randomised controlled trial focused on home safety and home exercise. The sample population comprised people aged 75 years and over, who had low vision and who were living in the community in New Zealand. The efficacy and cost effectiveness of a home safety programme and a home exercise programme were assessed, with falls being monitored for one year. Two occupational therapists delivered the home safety programme (n=100), and the exercise programme was provided by three physiotherapists (n=97); 98 participants received both of these programmes. Participants not randomised to the two intervention groups (n=96) received two social visits from a social visitor.

The home safety programme was modified for people with severe visual impairments and involved a home visit, the use of a modified version of the Westmead Home Safety Assessment, and discussion of recommendations. When equipment was recommended, this was followed by a second home visit where indicated. Adherence to the programme was evaluated after six months via a telephone interview.

Participants who engaged with the home safety programme had 41% fewer falls, and the intervention was more cost effective than the exercise programme for this group of people. The study suggested that an organisation seeking to reduce falls in older people with a visual impairment would 'do best by investing in a proved programme of home safety assessment and modification delivered by an occupational therapist' (Campbell et al 2005, p4).

A subsequent article based on the same research (**La Grow et al 2006**) set out to investigate whether the home safety assessment and modification programme success in reducing falls was related to the home hazards modification or modification of behaviour, or both. The type and location of the recommendations made by the occupational therapist were examined, together with the number and circumstances of falls experienced. The reduction in falls was found not to be limited to falls associated with an environmental hazard, and therefore the study concluded that the overall reduction in falls resulted from some mechanism in addition to the removal or modification of hazards or provision of new equipment.

The efficacy of environmental interventions in falls prevention was the subject of a systematic review by **Clemson et al (2008)**. This review focused on people aged 65 years and over living in the community, with an analysis of six trials that provided home environmental interventions as a single intervention (n=3,298). The primary outcome of interest was the rate of falls or proportion of fallers. Analysis identified there was a significant reduction in the risk of falls (21%) across all studies, with a greater reduction (39%) where the population was at high risk of falls (history of falling in past year, hospitalisation for a fall, severe visual impairment or functional decline). The review included a rating of intervention and determined that those of high intensity should meet 75% of four criteria. These criteria consisted of a comprehensive evaluation of hazard identification and priority-setting, taking into account both personal risk and environmental audit; the use of an assessment tool validated for the broad range of potential fall hazards; inclusion of formal or observational evaluation of the functional capacity of the person within the context of their environment; and provision of adequate follow-up and support for adaptations and modification. Studies that provided high-intensity intervention led by an occupational therapist significantly reduced the rate of falls.

Similar findings were found in a systematic review with inclusion criteria of studies of falls intervention programmes covering home hazard assessment with modification (4 studies), exercise and/or physical therapy (10 studies) or multifactorial intervention (12 studies) (**Costello and Edelstein 2008**). The evidence reviewed indicated that when targeted to older people at high risk of falls, home hazard assessment with modification may be beneficial in reducing falls.

A Cochrane review set out to establish which falls prevention interventions were effective for older people aged 65 years and over living in the community (**Gillespie et al 2012**). The review found that, overall, home safety assessment and modification interventions were effective in reducing the rate of falls (6 trials, n=4,208) and the risk of falling (7 trials, n=4,051). With respect to effectiveness, where there was a higher risk of falls (including those with severe visual impairment), home safety interventions were more effective in reducing the rate of falls. Risk of fracture was not significantly reduced, however. The review identified that there was some evidence that interventions led by an occupational therapist, compared with those not led by an occupational therapist, were more effective with respect to rate of falls and risk of falling.

An Italian quasi-randomised controlled trial assessed the role of a post-discharge home visit by an occupational therapist in reducing the risk of falling in females aged 60 years and over who had experienced a hip fracture (**Di Monaco et al 2008**). The usual multiprofessional intervention to prevent falls was delivered to all participants while in the rehabilitation hospital, but participants in the intervention group (n=45) received a home visit by an occupational therapist at a median point of 20 days post discharge; this was not provided to the control group (n=50). During the home visit, environmental hazards, activity of daily living behaviours, use of assistive devices and individualised targeted modifications were addressed. Falls were recorded by all participants and reported during a home visit taking place approximately six months after discharge. A significantly lower proportion of fallers were found in the intervention group following adjustment for observation length, Barthel Index scores assessed before the beginning of the observation period, and body height. The study reported that the reduction in the risk of sustaining one or more falls attributable to the home visit was 'remarkable' (adjusted absolute risk fell from 26% to 8.8%). The study, although relatively small and with some limitations in both methodology and sample, concluded that in a sample of older females discharged from a rehabilitation hospital following a first hip fracture, a single home visit by an occupational therapist significantly reduced their risk of falling.

A post-hoc analysis of the same study data examined the adherence to the home modification recommendations (**Di Monaco et al 2012**). Uncorrected environmental and behavioural factors significantly predicted fall occurrence for the participants in the high-risk group. These results were suggested as being indicative of a clear need to improve strategies to promote adherence.

The relationship between pre-discharge occupational therapy home assessments and prevalence of falls in the first month following discharge from a rehabilitation hospital was investigated in a prospective cohort study in Australia (**Johnston et al 2010**). The decision to undertake a home assessment was made by the treating occupational therapist based on clinical reasoning (n=223), and the number of falls for one month after discharge was recorded by all participants. The risk of falling one month after discharge was found to increase when considering all subjects not receiving a home assessment (n=119). Falls risk was mitigated by a home assessment for all diagnostic groups, with the exception of participants with neurological conditions, with a recommendation that diagnosis, falls risk and functional independence should be considered when deciding to carry out a home assessment.

The question of whether occupational therapy improves outcomes for people aged 60 years and over who are living independently was examined in a systematic review (**Steultjens et al 2004**). The search strategy included the primary outcome domain of incidence of falls and occupational therapy interventions, which included training of skills and advice and instruction regarding the use of assistive devices. The incidence of falling was measured in three randomised controlled trials, included in the review, which evaluated an intervention in which instructions in the use of assistive devices was combined with training of skills strategies. These provided some limited evidence for the efficacy of the intervention in decreasing falls incidence for people at high risk of falling. Strong evidence was identified within the review for the efficacy of advising on assistive devices as part of a home hazards assessment on functional ability.

Evidence overview
The evidence with respect to the effectiveness of the occupational therapist in home hazard assessments and interventions for people considered at high risk of falls (history of falling in past year, hospitalisation for a fall, severe visual impairment or functional decline) is both high quality and strong.

Keeping safe at home: reducing risk of falls

It is recommended that:

1. Service users who have fallen or are at risk of falls should be offered an occupational therapist-led home hazard assessment, including intervention and follow-up, to optimise functional activity and safety.   1A

   (Campbell et al 2005 [A]; Clemson et al 2008 [A]; Clemson et al 2004 [A]; Costello and Edelstein 2008 [B]; Gillespie et al 2012 [A]; La Grow et al 2006 [A]; Nikolaus and Bach 2003 [A]; Pighills et al 2011 [A])

Keeping safe at home: reducing risk of falls	
It is recommended that:	
2. Occupational therapists should offer home safety assessment and modification for older people with a visual impairment. *(Campbell et al 2005 [A]; Clemson et al 2008 [A]; Gillespie et al 2012 [A]; La Grow et al 2006 [A])*	1A
3. Occupational therapists should consider carrying out a pre- or post-discharge home assessment to reduce the risk of falls following discharge from an inpatient rehabilitation facility, taking into account the service user's falls risk, functional ability and diagnosis. *(Di Monaco et al 2012 [B]; Di Monaco et al 2008 [B]; Johnston et al 2010 [C])*	1B
4. Occupational therapists should offer service users who are living in the community advice, instruction and information on assistive devices as part of a home hazard assessment. *(Steultjens et al 2004 [B])*	1B

7.1.3 Potential impact of the recommendations

Outcomes sought:

- Service users make informed choices about how to manage the falls risks presented by their particular environments.

- Individuals are enabled to actively manage their risk of falls. Home hazards and behaviour are modifiable, but some medical falls risks are not.

Risks:

The context in which home hazard assessment and modification is provided should be considered. NICE (2013c) indicates that home hazard assessment and modification are not effective when completed as a standalone intervention, and should therefore be part of a multifactorial assessment and intervention.

Generalisability:

The evidence in this section has come from studies in which individuals are at least 60 years old, and therefore it can not be definitively generalised to younger people. The targeting of falls prevention to people at high risk (including those with visual impairment) has, however, been particularly highlighted, and these principles should be taken into account when working with younger people, in tandem with an individualised assessment and tailored approach to interventions.

The majority of the evidence originates from studies involving individuals living in the community, and specific research in hospitals or care homes is limited. One UK study carried out a cluster randomised control trial in care homes, with environmental modification as a component of the falls prevention programme (Dyer et al 2004); reduction in falls rates for the intervention groups did not reach statistical significance, and the authors' recommendations were reflective of the potential benefits of targeting people who have fallen or are at highest risk of falls.

Studies involving individuals with cognitive impairment or dementia are very limited, as these generally form exclusion criteria for participation. The potential for individuals with mild dementia to benefit from a home safety and exercise programme is, however, beginning to emerge, albeit in terms of acceptability rather than efficacy (Wesson et al 2013).

Social determinants of health:
It is important to note that assistive technology equipment provision in the UK is not universally a free provision, and the type of equipment prescribed or available is variable. Occupational therapists have to work within the eligibility requirements that may be stipulated by their local authority or organisation. The need to purchase equipment, the cost of which may be prohibitive for people on limited incomes, is an important factor to consider. Some individuals may not be able to make an informed choice about equipment or may not have easy access to obtain items independently. Occupational therapists therefore need to identify options for any equipment needs to be met and be mindful that several factors, of which lower economic status is an example, may influence the willingness of service users to accept help with home hazards (Yardley et al 2008).

7.2 Keeping active: reducing fear of falling

7.2.1 Introduction
Fear of falling has been suggested as being an umbrella term for 'fear, anxiety, loss of confidence and impaired perception of ability to walk safely without falling' (Parry et al 2013).

Fear may be experienced by people who have fallen and people who have never fallen and is experienced by up to half of older people living in the community (Zijlstra et al 2007). Fear of falling is, therefore, an important factor, particularly given its potentially detrimental consequences on an individual's lifestyle and activities.

The concept of self-efficacy, or the degree of confidence a person has in carrying out everyday activities without falling, is an important factor that needs to be considered in falls prevention and management.

> *"Loss or lack of confidence – I know if I fall there is a very high risk I will break a bone as I have osteoporosis. If I broke my hip there is a high chance I could die as a result. That makes you lack confidence."*
> *Rushcliffe 50+ Forum Health Group member*

The evidence and recommendations set out in this section can be considered within the framework of the NICE (2013c, p16) recommendation focusing on participation in falls prevention programmes:

> *Falls prevention programmes should also address potential barriers such as low self-efficacy and fear of falling, and encourage activity change as negotiated with the participant.* (Recommendation 1.1.9.1)

The evidence described has been reviewed in the context of the role of the occupational therapist within the delivery of this recommendation.

7.2.2 Evidence

The relationship between fear of falling and restricted activity is an area that has received attention within falls research, and studies included in the evidence have all been published within the last five years.

Boltz et al (2013) determined that fear of falling in people aged 70 years and over who were admitted to hospital resulted in activity restriction. The research, carried out in the United States of America, involved 41 participants with whom perceptions around mobility and physical activity and fear of falling were explored via semi-structured interviews and standardised measures. Participants who described themselves as depressed were more likely to describe fear of falling. Four themes were identified from the qualitative results, with a predominant response across those themes being activity restriction ('keeping still') versus self-direction ('use your common sense'). Fear of falling could potentially negatively influence mobility, physical activity and functional performance in older adults in hospital.

One theme from the qualitative results emphasised the importance of interpersonal factors, with participants highlighting the role of staff and their families in promoting safe mobility. The responsiveness and availability of staff in the hospital often influenced the level of physical activity. A reluctance to ask busy staff to help leading, on occasion, to 'stay[ing] put' (Boltz et al 2013, p7). Families were often described as facilitators and advocates in providing assistance that promoted independence. Restrictive environmental factors also emerged as a theme, exemplified by expressions from participants of perceived barriers to safe mobility and physical activity, including fall hazards. The need for staff to prioritise function-focused interventions within a context of an enabling philosophy emphasising independence and self-direction was identified. Although this study was undertaken in a hospital setting, the applicability of supporting staff and family in enabling physical activity, in the least restrictive way, is pertinent in all settings, such as in care homes, in home-based rehabilitation and as part of re-ablement.

A cross-sectional study in the Netherlands used a screening questionnaire to analyse self-reported information on a number of sociodemographic, health-related and psychosocial variables; levels of fear of falling; and avoidance of activity due to fear of falling (**Kempen et al 2009**). A total of 540 participants were included from a random selection of people aged 70 years and over living in the community. A number of correlations were identified: severe fear of falling correlated independently with being female, having limitations in activities of daily living, and one or more falls in the previous 6 months. Avoidance activity correlated independently with older age and limitations in activities of daily living.

An earlier study, also in the Netherlands, applied the Task Difficulty Homeostasis Theory to test out an assumption that the level of outdoor physical activity mediates the relationship between fear of falling and actual outdoor falls (**Wijlhuizen et al 2007**). The theory is founded on the principle that perceived task difficulty is related closely to the feeling of risk. This feeling represents an emotional response to a threat, such as fear of falling, and has consequences for related behaviour. The prospective study involved 1,752 people aged 65 years and older; questionnaires were completed about fear of falling outdoors and physical activity. Walking and bicycling were used as the indicators of outdoor physical activity. Participants who expressed a high fear of falling were more often low to moderately active; where there was a high fear of falls outdoors, participants restricted their outdoor physical activity to prevent an increase in falls in that environment. This research importantly confirmed that the incidence of falls alone as a measure is potentially limited, and the level of physical activity should also be taken into account.

"I had a fall on my front path and landed heavily on my knee. I have had a loss of confidence after my fall – although equipment helps, it does not restore your confidence."

Service user

The relationship of fear to depression, anxiety, activity level and activity restriction was the focus of a cohort study carried out by occupational therapy staff in the United States of America (**Painter et al 2012**). A 90-minute intervention delivered fall prevention information (including risk factors, fear of falling and home safety strategies), together with a semi-structured falls questionnaire and measures, including the Survey of Activities and Fear of Falling in the Elderly (SAFE). The intervention was undertaken with 99 participants aged 55 years and over who may or may not have experienced falls. The research found that activity level was correlated negatively with activity restriction, fear of falling, depression and anxiety. Furthermore, anxiety predicted both fear of falling and activity level. Clinical implications from this were that occupational therapy practitioners should assess for fear of falling when service users display anxiety and decreased motivation to perform functional activities.

"It's so important people listen to your fears and acknowledge them."

Rushcliffe 50+ Forum Health Group member

Schepens et al (2012) conducted a meta-analytical review to examine relationships between fall-related efficacy and measures of activity and participation of people aged 60 years and over living in the community. A strong positive relationship was identified between fall-related efficacy and activity on analysis of the 20 studies included in the review. The analysis indicated that both occupational-based activities (e.g. activities of daily living performance) and more basic performance skills (e.g. exercise to improve muscle strength) were affected by fall-related efficacy. The authors determined that the findings highlighted the important role of occupational therapists in assessing the link between fall-related efficacy and activity.

A systematic review examined the interventions to reduce fear of falling in older people living in the community (**Zijlstra et al 2007**). It concluded that home-based exercise, fall-related multifactorial programmes and community-based Tai Chi delivered in a group format had been effective in reducing fear of falling for this population. The article presented the perspective of fear of falling as being a response to a realistic threat but suggested that fear may also be associated with activities that could actually be performed safely. The potential social, mental and physical health adverse consequences of restricting activity were highlighted in the discussion, with the suggestion that 'the experience of performing activities safely may lead to greater falls self-efficacy and a realistic view of the risk of falling' (Zijlstra et al 2007, p614).

Evidence overview

The evidence on fear of falling highlights the integral link between fear and activity levels. Although reducing the number of falls may be a key outcome for falls prevention activities, the potential to restrict activity as a behavioural response to fear of falling can be to the detriment of activities of daily living and occupational engagement. People have different attitudes and levels of tolerance to risk. The occupational therapist therefore has a valuable role in working with service users, caregivers, family and friends to achieve a balance of risk and activity.

Keeping active: reducing fear of falling

It is recommended that:

5. Occupational therapists should explore with service users whether fear of falling may be restricting activity, both in and outside the home, and include the promotion of occupational activity within individualised intervention plans.   1C

    (Boltz et al 2013 [C]; Kempen et al 2009 [C]; Painter et al 2012 [C]; Wijlhuizen et al 2007 [C])

6. Occupational therapists should listen to an individual's subjective views about their falls risk, alongside using objective functionally based outcomes, to determine the influence of fear of falling on the service user's daily life.   1B

    (Schepens et al 2012 [B]; Wijlhuizen et al 2007 [C])

7. Occupational therapists should seek ways of enabling service users to minimise the risk of falling when performing chosen activities, wherever possible, as this may improve confidence and enable realistic risk taking.   1B

    (Wijlhuizen et al 2007 [C]; Zijlstra et al 2007 [B])

8. Occupational therapists should facilitate caregivers, family and friends to adopt a positive approach to risk.   1C

    (Boltz et al 2013 [C])

7.2.3 Potential impact of the recommendations

Outcomes sought:
- Occupational therapists are aware of those individuals restricting activity due to fear of falling and can therefore consider intervention strategies.

- Service users confidently engage in their daily activities and occupations, with a realistic understanding of any potential risk of falling.

- Caregivers are confident in allowing the service user to take appropriate and relevant risk.

Risks:
Reducing fear may increase activity, which conversely may increase falls and potentially lead to individuals taking risks that are beyond their balance capabilities.

Generalisability:
The evidence included studies within the home, in the outside environment and in the hospital setting. Fear of falling is likely to impact on activity within any context or

environment, and the recommendations can therefore potentially be translated to all settings. It is acknowledged, however, that some members of the multidisciplinary team may be more circumspect about promoting positive risk-taking, for example in the acute hospital environment compared with the familiar environment of the service user's home.

Social determinants of health:
Fear of falling can affect activities of daily living and occupational engagement. Reducing fear can contribute to maximising individual capacity and control over life and the potential to impact positively on preventing associated ill health such as anxiety.

7.3 Falls management: making it meaningful

7.3.1 Introduction
The delivery of occupational therapy services is underpinned by the principles of working in partnership with service users, putting them at the centre of practice, and upholding their right to make choices about the care they receive (COT 2010).

Person-centred care is a complex concept with many dimensions, but the evidence on the meaning of person-centred care has identified common principles (de Silva 2014). The principles most pertinent to falls prevention and management include:

- 'Recognising the person's individuality and specificity.

- Taking a holistic approach to assessing needs and providing care (which may include families and recognising social and environmental factors as part of a biopsychosocial perspective).

- Seeing the patient as an expert about their own health and care; recognising autonomy and thus sharing power and responsibility, including enablement and activation in decisions about care.

- Ensuring that services are accessible, flexible to individual needs and easy to navigate.'

(de Silva 2014, p9)

Recommendations for promoting the engagement of older people in activities to prevent falls were developed in a project undertaken by the Prevention of Falls Network Earth (ProFaNE) (Yardley et al 2007). Based on a literature review, including studies of older people's views, clinical expertise and subsequent consensus, six recommendations were outlined. The recommendations of particular relevance here are the importance of tailoring interventions to the individual's specific situation and values and ensuring an understanding about the benefits of falls interventions.

> "The problem with the term 'risk assessment' is that it implies all risks are the same, and they aren't. Some things you might try and do could be very risky, others hardly risky at all."
>
> Rushcliffe 50+ Forum Health Group member

A sample of 66 older people's perceptions of falls prevention advice was reported in a qualitative study. Participants commonly considered falls prevention advice as being useful in principle but not personally relevant or appropriate. Falls were associated with a potential threat to autonomy and identity, and participants identified that falls risk and prevention should be portrayed more constructively (Yardley et al 2006).

The evidence base for multifactorial interventions is strong (NICE 2013c), but the effect of this will be negated, and falls prevention and management will not be effective, if service users decline to participate.

The evidence reviewed and recommendations set out in this section can be considered within the framework of the NICE (2013c, p15) recommendation for encouraging the participation of older people in falls prevention programmes:

> *Healthcare professionals involved in the assessment and prevention of falls should discuss what changes a person is willing to make to prevent falls.* (Recommendation 1.1.9.1)

The evidence reviewed has been considered specifically with regard to the role of the occupational therapist within the delivery of this recommendation.

7.3.2 Evidence

A number of sources of evidence explored the psychosocial issues, motivational factors and barriers associated with the engagement of adults in falls prevention activities.

Nyman's (2011) overview of theory and studies focused on psychosocial factors influencing older people's participation in physical activity interventions aimed at preventing falls. Factors affecting participation were described by the theory of planned behaviour framework. Three variables were of particular note: (1) the individual's attitude towards the behaviour, in this context interpreted as perceived falls risk and belief about whether falls can be prevented; (2) the views of others, the subjective norm, can influence engagement, with favourable opinions from significant others being important in accepting activities; and (3) perceived behavioural control, which in respect of falls is related to confidence and fear of falling. Where perceived behavioural control is low, an individual's fear may reduce their likelihood of participating. Knowledge was also identified as important in influencing engagement in falls prevention interventions, but in isolation knowledge was not a sufficient motivator. Understanding the reasons for falling and recognising external and preventable causes (extrinsic risk factors) were identified as particularly important when encouraging engagement to prevent secondary falls. Older people are more likely to carry out falls prevention activities when they 'perceive that the activities will afford positive benefits and that [those] benefits are highly likely to occur' (Nyman 2011, p48). The review provides evidence that it is not only what is done in falls prevention interventions, but also how it is approached, that will influence engagement and active participation.

> "It's so important people have a chance to express what they want, what they need – not to be 'done to' but to be listened to and heard."
>
> Rushcliffe 50+ Forum Health Group member

A qualitative study carried out by **de Groot and Fagerström (2011)** explored the factors that both motivated and presented barriers to participating in a local group exercise intervention, through semi-structured interviews with ten older people. The theoretical framework for this research was the 'motivational equation', and the findings presented highlighted the importance of the perceptions of the individual. Specifically, the researchers identified from their analysis four factors within the motivational equation: (1) perceived chance of success (including confidence in oneself, control over and perceptions of one's health); (2) perceived importance of the goal (knowledge, a desire to 'get better' and preferences regarding group or individual intervention); (3) perceived costs; and (4) inclination to remain sedentary. In the context of support from health professionals, most of the participants in the study suggested that it was the duty of the health professional to inform service users about the benefits of the intervention, in this case exercise, to give them the 'push' to get started (de Groot and Fagerström 2011, p157). Although this study focused particularly on exercise groups in Norway, the motivational model confirmed the importance of health professionals in identifying the motivating factors and barriers for each person.

Falls are a complex health issue and not limited to physical factors. A Canadian study recruited eight volunteers from a retired older population who had fallen (but not sustained an injury requiring medical attention) within the past 12 months (**Gopaul and Connelly 2012**). The study investigated how knowledge of one's own fall risk influenced self-reported behaviours and beliefs about falls. A mix of qualitative interviews, questionnaires and assessment measures were administered. The intervention consisted of tailored education, based on the individual's estimated risk of falling and their own home environment. A personalised home safety booklet was also provided. The authors found that an individual's awareness about falls increased over time during the study, but a recurring barrier was that participants did not want to admit their susceptibility to falling and hence avoided engagement in fall prevention activities.

The importance of involving service users in the decision-making process with respect to falls prevention interventions was identified within a critical literature review undertaken by **Wilkins et al (2003)**. The review considered the evidence on the effectiveness of community-based occupational therapy education and functional training programmes for older adults. Of the three studies included in the review that were fall related, two identified that not all home modifications recommended were implemented or followed up (Clemson et al 1999, Cummings et al 1999). The ability to take ownership of ideas and retain control, together with the ability to explore options and choices, were found to be strong influences in acceptance and implementation of home modification recommendations.

> *"People are all different – how they express this [risk of falls] will also be different – some will need encouragement to do more, others may need holding back a bit."*
>
> *Rushcliffe 50+ Forum Health Group member*

A more recent study likewise highlighted that service users should be offered choices and options. **Currin et al (2012)** aimed to identify the uptake of home modifications recommended by occupational therapists in a sample of 80 people aged over 60 years living in the community who had experienced a recent fall. The intrinsic and extrinsic factors that might predict the uptake of recommendations was also investigated. Participants in this cohort study nested within a larger randomised control trial all received an initial joint occupational therapist and physiotherapist home visit. The environmental assessment undertaken by the occupational therapist used the Falls Prevention Environmental Audit – Community Tool, which covers eight categories (bathrooms and toilets, bedrooms, floor surfaces, furniture, lighting, mobility aids, passageways and external areas), each with prompt questions. Usual practice was followed for referrals for equipment or modifications. Fifty-five per cent of the recommendations made had been completed by six months. Adherence was identified as a 'complex interplay' of intrinsic and extrinsic factors. Frailer individuals (those with more comorbidities) were more likely to accept modifications, and the coexistence of depression or psychological distress had a negative impact on the uptake of home visit recommendations. Interestingly, adherence was also influenced by the site and type of recommendation and who was responsible for its implementation: recommendations requiring external provider action were more likely to be completed than those where implementation depended on the service user or family members. Although potentially having site-specific features related to the Australian system of the provision of equipment and adaptations, the importance of occupational therapists taking into account a range of factors and giving the service user maximum control is reinforced. As identified by the authors, 'The full potential of an occupational therapy home environmental audit recommendations will be achieved only if recommended modifications are actually implemented' (Currin et al 2012, p90).

Ballinger and Clemson (2006) undertook a qualitative study in Australia that explored the views of 11 participants (median age 76 years) about the most and least useful aspects of the falls intervention programme in which they had participated. The programme, entitled 'Stepping On', was multifactorial and consisted of seven sessions, including topics such as benefits of exercise and identifying home hazards (Clemson et al 2004). Four themes emerged from the analysis of the semi-structured interviews that took place three months after the programme: identity; salience of interventions ('meaning attributed to the various components of the programme'); social experience; and consequences of participation.

Participants reflected on both the content and the process of the programme, identifying some aspects of the programme that they perceived as less useful or relevant to them. Medication management, home hazards and footwear discussions were identified by men as being potentially valuable but not relevant to them. Accounts from participants also referred to the variety of models of learning and teaching; at times the researchers noted these accounts were divergent.

The theme of 'consequences of participation' highlighted that participants rarely referred to a decrease in the likelihood of a fall. Outcomes important to the individuals were changes in performance, skills or attributes. An increase in confidence was the major psychological benefit identified. The study concluded that the perceived positive benefits were broader than preventing falls and had a 'connectedness to the more intrinsic values of independence and issues of wellbeing' (Ballinger and Clemson 2006, p269).

A randomised controlled trial in Australia aimed to assess the effectiveness of a targeted multiple interventions falls prevention programme in a subacute hospital (**Haines et al 2006, Haines et al 2004, Stern and Jayasekara 2009**). Although this study recruited adults of all ages, ranging from 38 to 99 years, the average age was 80 years. One element was an education programme consisting of individual sessions of up to 30 minutes twice a week. This included general information on falls and fall-prevention strategies, goal-setting and review, a quiz, fall risk assessment and booklet. The intervention was recommended by the hospital occupational therapists but conducted by a research occupational therapist. In the study subgroup analysis of 226 participants, there was a significantly lower incidence of falls in the intervention group (n=115) than in the control group (n=111). This finding was applicable to participants who received the education-only intervention and those who received the education and other interventions. Participants were asked to complete an evaluation survey; the majority of those responding (64 of 115) indicated that they agreed or strongly agreed that the written education material was easy to understand, the information was new, and their falls prevention behaviour had been modified as a result. The authors indicated that although it could not be concluded with certainty that the education programme was solely responsible for the reduction in falls, the findings indicated that an education

package was effective and should be incorporated as part of a multifactorial prevention programme for subacute hospital inpatients.

The presentation of falls prevention information can make a difference to the potential for uptake, and this aspect of falls prevention was explored in an evaluative study undertaken by **Nyman et al (2011)**. The way that older people were represented and how information was presented on 33 fall-prevention websites was evaluated using discourse analysis principles. This identified three potential positions for older people: the passive recipient, the rational learner and the empowered decision-maker. The falls-prevention advice offered was viewed as being unlikely to be effective, given that many websites were not engaging, representing older people as passive and inert. The importance of projecting an image that would be congruent with positive self-identity and promotion of self-management, in line with the recommendations made by ProFaNE (Yardley et al 2007), was evident. The authors provided suggestions for occupational therapists to ensure that falls prevention advice is written, whether for information leaflets or the internet, in a way that empowers older people.

Alternative modes of delivering falls prevention information were a focus of a two-group randomised controlled trials undertaken in Australia (**Hill et al 2009**). This research evaluated the effectiveness of falls prevention information delivered to older people in hospital, comparing DVD-delivered education (n=49) with a written workbook (n=51). The control group received no education (n=131), and their data were collected during an initial quasi-experimental phase of the study. No significant difference was established between the two education groups with respect to self-perceived falls risk or knowledge of falls. The DVD group, however, had a higher proportion of participants who were strongly motivated to prevent themselves falling, compared with the workbook group. The research indicated that multimedia offers alternatives to traditional written approaches for providing health-related information. This may facilitate better uptake of information and have an influence on perceptions and motivation to participate.

A randomised controlled trial in Sweden evaluated the effectiveness of a high-intensity functional exercise programme in reducing falls (**Rosendahl et al 2008**). The setting was residential care (nine facilities); the 191 participants were aged 65 years or over. The control activity programme was developed by occupational therapists and consisted of themed activities performed while sitting, such as watching films, reading, singing and conversation. The High-Intensity Functional Exercise Programme (HIFE) used in the intervention group did not significantly reduce the fall rate or the proportion of participants who sustained a fall when all participants were compared during the six-month follow-up period. Analysis revealed that the subgroup of participants who improved their balance in the intervention group had a lower fall rate than the control group. This study was particularly interesting in that the control activity programme had an effect on physical function (determined using the Berg Balance Scale), potentially through 'the impact of social stimulation, meaningful activities, or transferring to another location in the facility' (Rosendahl et al 2008, p73).

The importance of meaningful falls prevention interventions was evidenced through the Lifestyle Integrated Functional Exercise (LiFE) approach in a three-arm randomised controlled trial undertaken by **Clemson et al (2012)** in Australia. This built on the outcomes of an earlier pilot study (**Clemson et al 2010**). The LiFE approach, which was developed by two occupational therapists, a gerontologist and a physiotherapist, involved teaching well-researched principles of balance and strength training. These were integrated into balance and strength strategies and applied in individualised daily activities meaningful to the individual. There were four balance strategies: reducing base of support; moving to the limits of sway; shifting weight from foot to foot; and stepping over objects. An activity (such as working at the kitchen worktop) might initially involve a tandem stand (heel-to-toe stand), subsequently upgrading over time to carry out the activity standing on one leg, hence reducing the base of support. The principle involved providing activities that could be carried out in the course of everyday life, potentially a number of times a day, and also could be upgraded to be more challenging. A similar principle was applied to strategies to improve strength. A LiFE manual supported the individualised programme.

A total of 107 participants were randomised to the LiFE programme. The other two arms of the study comprised a structured programme of exercises carried out three times a week (n=105) and a sham control programme of gentle exercise (n=105). Participants were aged 70 years or more and had a history of falls in the previous six months. The LiFE group resulted in a clinically significant 31% reduction in the rate of falls compared with the control programme, and the structured exercise group showed a 19% non-significant reduction in the rate of falls compared with the control group. Function and participation were greater in the LiFE programme, and adherence was better at 12 months. The LiFE programme was viewed as providing a real alternative to traditional exercise, being based on function and with outcomes of 'increased energy to do more tasks, improved functioning during activities and enhanced participation in daily life' (Clemson et al 2012, p6).

The potential motivational value in promoting participation in occupations that are meaningful to the individual and take place in the everyday environment was highlighted within a systematic review (**Pritchard et al 2013**). Inclusion criteria included people aged 65 years and over in the post-discharge period from a hospital or an emergency department visit. The review identified that longitudinal studies have shown that long-term adherence to falls prevention activities, such as exercise, is often poor. Motivation can be a barrier, and the authors suggested that programmes such as LiFE, which are underpinned by embedding activity into everyday routines, could be a key principle in promoting uptake.

Evidence overview
Occupational therapists should maximise the engagement of the service user in falls management interventions, taking into consideration the service user's motivation, beliefs and knowledge.

A key message to be incorporated into falls prevention and management interventions is a focus on the potential benefits to the individual of interventions to improve mobility, independence and active participation, as distinct to the language used within the professional arena of 'reducing the incidence of falls' or 'decreasing the risk of falls'. Service users should be made aware of the potential implications of falling, but occupational therapists should highlight the positive outcomes rather than the negative connotations associated with falls.

Meaningful activity can be linked integrally with motivation. Physical activity which can be incorporated into daily lifestyles is more likely to be sustainable; there is a key role here for occupational therapists given this functional approach. The value of such an occupational and activity-based approach is supported by the high-quality research by Clemson and colleagues. Although the primary research for the LiFE approach was undertaken in Australia (Clemson et al 2012, Clemson et al 2010), potentially it is easily translatable to the United Kingdom.

Falls management: making it meaningful	
It is recommended that:	
9. Occupational therapists should share knowledge and understanding of falls prevention and management strategies with the service user. This should provide personally relevant information and take account of the service user's individual fall risk factors, lifestyle and preferences. *(Ballinger and Clemson 2006 [C]; de Groot and Fagerström 2011 [C]; Haines et al 2006 [C]; Haines et al 2004 [B]; Stern and Jayasekara 2009 [B])*	1B
10. Occupational therapists should take into account the service user's perceptions and beliefs regarding their ability, and personal motivation, which may influence participation in falls intervention. *(de Groot and Fagerström 2011 [C]; Gopaul and Connelly 2012 [D]; Nyman 2011 [C])*	1C
11. Occupational therapists should maximise the extent to which the service user feels in control of the falls intervention. *(Currin et al 2012 [C]; Wilkins et al 2003 [C])*	1C
12. Occupational therapists should support the engagement of the service user in identifying the positive benefits of falls intervention. *(Ballinger and Clemson 2006 [C]; Nyman 2011 [C])*	1C
13. Falls prevention and management information should be available in different formats and languages to empower and engage all populations (e.g. web-based support, written information leaflets). *(Hill et al 2009 [B]; Nyman et al 2011 [C])*	1B
14. Physical and social activity, as a means of reducing an individual's risk of falls and their adverse consequences, should be encouraged and supported through the use of activities meaningful to the individual. *(Rosendahl et al 2008 [B])*	1B
15. Activities to improve strength and balance should be incorporated into daily activities and occupations that are meaningful to the individual, to improve and encourage longer-term participation in falls prevention interventions. *(Clemson et al 2012 [A]; Clemson et al 2010 [B]; Pritchard et al 2013 [B])*	1A

7.3.3 Potential impact of the recommendations

Outcomes sought:

- Service users continue to engage in occupational life roles while understanding and contributing to reducing their individual risk of falls.

- Uptake and adherence of falls prevention programmes is improved, thus contributing to reducing the incidence and risk of falls.

- Service users have choice and control over what happens and can recognise the potential for positive outcomes in terms of health and wellbeing, independence and social roles.

- Falls risk is reduced by incorporating exercise into daily life activities.

- Information and resources on preventing and managing falls are available in a range of accessible formats that empower the service user.

- Cost efficiency for NHS and social care providers in service delivery.

Risks:

One of the risks of implementing the engagement and active participation recommendations above is an increased risk of falls. The rationale here is that older people often reduce their risk of falling by reducing their physical activity (Wijlhuizen et al 2010); therefore, if they are encouraged to become more physically active through engagement in falls prevention activities, they may conversely increase their risk (Wijlhuizen et al 2008). Some association between the risk of falls increasing with more active participation in rehabilitation has been identified (Czernuszenko and Członkowska 2009, Lee and Stokic 2008).

Generalisability:

Evidence within the area of active participation and engagement was based on research or reviews with participants who were, with the exception of one study, aged 60 years or over. Most studies did not include participants with cognitive impairment.

It is suggested, however, that the fundamental nature of person-centred principles and individualised intervention cuts across all ages and clinical conditions and enables these recommendations to be directly relevant to occupational therapy falls prevention and management with all adults.

Social determinants of health:

A person-centred approach to engagement is more likely to ensure that the needs of all populations are considered and enable participation of even the most vulnerable adults in falls intervention, maximising individual capacity and control over life.

8 Service users' perspectives of falls

Valuable perspectives of the meaning of a fall were gained from service users attending the pre-consultation meeting and participating in the guideline consultation. Quotes from the service users are included, where relevant, in Section 7; others are provided here.

The personal impact of falls on an individual can be significant:

> *"Falls mean a loss of independence and a fear of doing more damage to myself (I have fallen and broken my wrist). Also embarrassment about unsteadiness and poor balance."*
>
> *Younger adult diagnosed with Gluten Ataxia*

> *"A loss of independence for some older people, fearful of what might happen to them."*
>
> *Service user*

> *"You have to accept what is realistic – some things you may not be able to do any more. But that can be very difficult, especially when you are only in your 60s."*
>
> *Rushcliffe 50+ Forum Health Group member*

> *"It is the fact a fall is accidental and unexpected – it is a shock."*
>
> *Rushcliffe 50+ Forum Health Group member*

> *"Pain, broken bones and anxiety about who was going to look after me, feed me etc."*
>
> *Service user*

> *"The problem is that it's everything that might not be working so well – like your hands so you can't pull yourself up so easily, then that makes you less steady."*
>
> *Rushcliffe 50+ Forum Health Group member*

> *"When I was really unwell I had over ten falls a day. This was often terrifying. I felt disabled and scared of injury. I had many cuts and bruises and was embarrassed to be in public so stopped at home, unable to work or socialise."*
>
> *Younger adult with multiple sclerosis*

College of Occupational Therapists

QUEEN MARGARET UNIVERSITY LRC

51

9 Implementation of the guideline

This practice guideline aims to support occupational therapists to take the most appropriate action when working with adults who have fallen, are at risk of falling, or are fearful of falling.

Familiarisation with the guideline document will be an important first step for individual practitioners and their managers. It is therefore imperative that occupational therapists and managers working in this clinical area take responsibility to review the guideline recommendations within the context of their practice.

Bringing the guideline to the attention of colleagues within the multidisciplinary team and service commissioners should also be a priority.

A further action to facilitate implementation must be for lead therapists to consider the levers and barriers within their local organisation and culture that may have an impact on any changes that may be necessary to practice. Section 9.2 identifies potential barriers that may be applicable, and Section 9.3 describes resources to facilitate implementation.

9.1 Dissemination and promotion

Awareness and implementation of this practice guideline are important if it is to influence and have an impact on occupational therapy practice.

Following publication in December 2014, the full practice guideline has been made available to download freely from the College of Occupational Therapists' website and can additionally be accessed via the COTSS-Older People web pages.

The guideline has been promoted to its key target audience of occupational therapists and to relevant others using professional networks and publications, internet and social media channels.

9.2 Organisational and financial barriers

The recommendations stated within this guideline document are intended to facilitate occupational therapy staff to contribute effectively to those outcomes important to the service user and to the delivery of falls prevention and management services.

The occupational therapist's individualised approach, which takes into account the person, the environment and their occupation (Law et al 1996), is an important facilitator in the effective implementation of the recommendations.

It is recognised, however, that there will be potential barriers, both organisational and financial, that may influence application of the recommendations. It is important that occupational therapists take these into account when implementing this guideline.

9.2.1 Organisational barriers

There are a number of potential organisational barriers that may impact on an occupational therapist's ability to implement the recommendations within this guideline. The most likely barriers were identified via consensus agreement of the clinical experts in the GDG:

- In some organisations, policy means generic or unqualified or lesser-skilled staff complete home hazard checklist risk assessments.

- Some services operate with strong drivers for high levels of turnover or there are limits on the number or duration of sessions to deliver fall prevention and management interventions. Working with individuals with fear of falling may require a number of contacts to provide individualised intervention; the need for flexibility may be particularly evident when service users require more assistance with expressing or determining their wishes, such as people with sensory impairment, learning difficulties, cognitive impairment or dementia.

- Some organisations are mandated to achieve a reduction in fall rates with a formulaic or process-driven approach to falls intervention that focuses on reporting falls and their adverse consequences.

- Some services perceive falls as separate to their specialty or not part of their core remit.

- Occupational therapists may not feel sufficiently skilled in working with the specific needs of service users who are visually impaired. There may be a training requirement with both organisational and resource implications and the need for access to visual impairment specialists.

- There may be a lack of financial resources to facilitate home assessment from a rehabilitation or acute setting, such as transport of the service user with the occupational therapist.

9.2.2 Cost-effectiveness and financial barriers

Falls, and their consequences, have significant financial costs for health and social care services (NICE 2013b, Tian et al 2013).

The cost-effectiveness of providing falls prevention has been investigated, and a small number of economic evaluations, not all of which met the guideline inclusion criteria, were identified via the NHS Economic Evaluation Database search. The heterogeneous focus of such studies means their outcomes should be interpreted with caution.

An economic evaluation of a randomised controlled trial providing a multidisciplinary programme (including occupational therapy) in a day hospital in the UK indicated an association with fewer falls but was more costly than usual care (Irvine et al 2010). A mean cost of £349, which included occupational therapy review and home visit (although not used by all participants), was identified for the prevention programme, but additional costs resulted in a mean incremental cost of £578 for the intervention. The estimated incremental cost-effectiveness ratio was £3,320 per fall averted. Cost-effectiveness was, however, identified in less than 40% of the simulations.

Campbell et al (2005) examined cost-effectiveness ratios and undertook a sensitivity analysis as part of their randomised controlled trial of a home safety programme, in New Zealand, for people with a visual impairment. Resource use and unit costs for the intervention led by occupational therapy were included, with details broken down into training costs, recruitment and programme delivery. The mean programme cost per person was equivalent to £117, with the cost per fall prevented calculated at £234. This study identified that falls can be prevented at a cost but, by applying a targeted approach, the associated costs could be reduced.

The actual costs of implementing the occupational therapy components of multifactorial falls prevention and management interventions are influenced by many factors. Services may be delivered across a wide range of health, social care and other settings, with variables associated with local workforce structure, service design and community equipment policy. Distinguishing costs related directly to falls prevention and management may be more difficult to estimate outside of specific falls prevention services or detailed cost-effectiveness or economic evaluation research.

Finance-related barriers that occupational therapists may experience in the implementation of the recommendations were identified, via consensus of the clinical experts in the GDG, as potentially including:

- Failure to commission or fund occupational therapists to deliver fall prevention and management interventions.

- Lack of funding for the provision of equipment and assistive devices recommended following assessment, from statutory services or individual service users.

- Limited resources to provide information and materials for service users in a range of accessible presentation styles, particularly if using multimedia and technologically supported formats.

The overall most critical resource required to implement these guideline recommendations is undoubtedly the availability of occupational therapists within the multidisciplinary team. Although generic working may be a driving force in some services, the evidence demonstrates the effective contribution of the occupational therapist in the delivery of multifactorial assessment and interventions for the prevention and management of falls.

9.3 Implementation resources

Three core implementation resources are available to support this practice guideline.

9.3.1 Quick reference guide

The quick reference guide is intended to be used by practitioners as an easily accessible reminder of the recommendations for intervention. It should ideally be used once the practitioner has read the full guideline document. This is important to ensure an appreciation and understanding of how the recommendations were developed and their context.

The quick reference guide includes the following:

- List of recommendations, their strengths and the quality of evidence leading to their development.

- Background to clinical condition.

- Occupational therapy role.

9.3.2 Audit form

It is recommended that occupational therapists participate in audit of fall prevention services, including auditing against the recommendations in this guideline.

The audit form for this guideline provides a standard template for individual occupational therapists or services to audit and review their current interventions against the individual recommendations. The aim is to encourage a reflection on current practice and, where this does not follow the recommendations, to consider the clinical reasoning in place to support decisions.

A baseline assessment conducted using the audit tool can be repeated to enable review of progress on actions identified from the audit. It can be useful to undertake a routine audit every 1–2 years to monitor ongoing compliance.

The audit form, although initially providing a tool for use within an individual or service context, offers the potential for future benchmarking. The COTSS-Older People will explore, within their business planning process, the feasibility and options for undertaking a wider comparative analysis over the next two years.

9.3.3 Continuing professional development session

A set of PowerPoint slides and supporting documentation provides the resources for an individual or service to conduct a continuing professional development session focused on the practice guideline. The learning outcomes for the session are to:

- Explore aspects of the evidence-based guideline/recommendations in relation to current practice.

- Develop an understanding of the importance of using an evidence-based guideline to inform practice.

- Explore and develop an understanding of how to use the College of Occupational Therapists' audit tool for the evidence-based recommendations.

The slides can also be valuable in increasing awareness about the guideline and can be tailored to meet local needs.

In addition to the audit form, which is most likely to be used by services, a reflective practice template is available for occupational therapists to review their own practice.

A feedback form is available to comment on the guideline and implementation resources to the College of Occupational Therapists.

The quick reference guide, audit form and continuing professional development session resources are available as separate documents. These can be downloaded, together with the full guideline document, from the publications section of the College of Occupational Therapists' website, and can also be accessed via the COTSS-Older People web pages.

10 Recommendations for future research

The review of the evidence identified occupational therapy primary research, predominantly with respect to home hazard and modification with older people, but in the context of certain population and setting exclusions.

'The effectiveness of occupation-focused interventions continues to be the major priority identified by occupational therapists for research activity' (COT 2007, p12). Establishing effectiveness is linked closely to the use of standardised assessments and outcome measures in the provision of services and to cost-effectiveness studies that support the commissioning of occupation-focused services (COT 2013a).

The GDG recommends a number of potential topics where further research could be focused.

- Effective falls prevention and management strategies for:
  - Adults aged under 60 years.
  - Individuals with cognitive impairment or living with dementia, and their carers.
  - Service users with mental health needs in community and inpatient settings.
  - People with a learning disability.
- Occupational therapy-specific fall prevention programmes (LiFE, Stepping On) within the UK context.
- Uptake of home hazard advice and implementation of occupational therapy-specific recommendations.
- Meaningful activity-based interventions and engagement of residents in care homes to reduce risk of falls.
- Occupational therapy, assistive technology and falls.
- Occupational therapy-specific assessment tools and outcome measures for falls.
- Use of psychological approaches by occupational therapists in the management of falls.
- Occupational therapy-led education and training programmes in the prevention and management of falls in care homes.
- Occupational therapy-led education for service users, carers and staff working with adults who are at risk of falling.

> 'I would like to see more guidelines about helping carers of people with dementia, especially for those who care alone, as when they are doing something in another room than the person with dementia like cooking and the person with dementia has been seated in a chair with no support at the side, they can fall.'
>
> Chairman, Carers in Hucknall

The GDG endorses the research recommendations identified by the NICE clinical guideline on falls, but in particular those relating to:

- Identifying which components of multifactorial interventions are important in different settings and among different patient groups.
- Identifying cost-effective components of multifactorial programmes for particular groups of older people in different settings (NICE 2013c, p186).
- Environmental adaptations in inpatient units.
- Falls prevention intervention effectiveness in inpatient units (NICE 2013c, pp252–253).

11 Updating the guideline

The National Executive Committee of the COTSS-Older People is responsible for ensuring future review of this guideline and will provide a focal point for any feedback received on the guideline following its publication, and relevant new evidence identified by the Falls Clinical Forum.

Occupational therapists have a continuous personal responsibility to keep abreast of evidence specific to occupational therapy. Members of the COTSS-Older People will also be made aware of any significant developments in evidence relevant to the guideline that may be identified before its formal review. Dissemination of information will primarily be achieved via the COTSS-Older People web pages, newsletter distributions, and an update on the evidence base presented at their annual conference.

The wider membership of the British Association of Occupational Therapists will be made aware of any significant developments in the evidence base via the publication *OTnews*.

This practice guideline is scheduled for update by 2020. The review date, however, may be brought forward if there is significant new evidence that may impact on practice.

Information about the COTSS-Older People is available at:
http://www.cot.co.uk/cotss-older-people/cot-ss-older-people.

Appendix 1: Guideline Development Group

Kate Robertson (Project Lead)
- MSc, PGCert (Falls and Osteoporosis), DipCOT
- Consultant Therapist in Falls Prevention, Nottinghamshire Healthcare NHS Trust, Nottinghamshire
- Associate Lecturer, University of Derby, Derby
- COTSS-Older People: Member

Shelley Crossland
- BSc (Hons) Occupational Therapy
- Occupational Therapist, Mental Health Services for Older People, Leicestershire Partnership NHS Trust, Leicestershire
- COTSS-Older People: Member

Jo Doubleday
- BSc (Hons) Occupational Therapy
- Independent Occupational Therapist
- Specialises in writing and delivering falls prevention training programmes in care homes and for Local Authority Staff
- COTSS-Older People: Member

Dr Judi Edmans
- PhD, MPhil, DipCOT, FCOT
- Senior Research Fellow, University of Nottingham, Nottingham
- COTSS-Older People: Research and Development Lead (to October 2013)
- COTSS-Neurological Practice: Newsletter Editor
- Royal College of Physicians Intercollegiate Working Party for Stroke (National Clinical Guidelines for Stroke): Member

Tessa Fiddes
- PGCert (Advanced Practice), DipCOT
- Team Leader/Falls Clinical Specialist Occupational Therapist, Older People's Medicine, Norfolk and Norwich University Hospitals NHS Foundation Trust, Norwich
- COTSS-Older People: Member

Lianne McInally
- MBA Public Services Management, BSc (Hons) Occupational Therapy
- Falls Advanced Occupational Therapist, Falls Service NHS Lanarkshire currently seconded to National Project Lead, Up and About in Care Homes – The management of falls and fractures in Care Homes for Older People Improvement Project
- COTSS-Older People: Falls Clinical Forum Co-Lead (Guideline Development Group member from August 2013)

Catherina Nolan
- MSc, BSc (Hons) Occupational Therapy
- Head Occupational Therapist, Medicine for the Elderly and General Medicine, Imperial College Healthcare NHS Trust, London
- COTSS-Older People: Chair

Zoe Foan
- Clinical Specialist for Older People, Virgin Care (Surrey) and COTSS-Older People: Falls Clinical Forum Co-Lead, was involved as a member of the guideline development group for the proposal and scope development (January–July 2013)

Appendix 2: Acknowledgements

The GDG would like to thank all those who have contributed to the development of this practice guideline.

1. Service user reference groups

Rushcliffe 50+ Forum Health Group, Nottinghamshire

Mrs Sue Knowles, chair of Rushcliffe 50+ Forum Health Group, is acknowledged for her assistance in facilitation of the consultation with members of the group

National Osteoporosis Society Norwich and Nottingham groups

2. Service users (individuals)

Invaluable views and comments on the draft guideline during the consultation period, were provided by the following individual service users who have personal experience of falling:

- Gladys Bombek
- Ann Burne
- Jim Radburn
- Tony Wilde
- Ken Williams

3. Stakeholder reference group

- Tim Chesser, British Orthopaedic Association Trauma Group
- Catherine Dennison, Head of Research – Health and Wellbeing, and Suzy England, Occupational Therapy and Sight Loss Consultant, Thomas Pocklington Trust
- Lisa Field, Consultant Radiographer, Mid Yorkshire NHS Trust, on behalf of the Society and College of Radiographers
- Joe Godden, Professional Officer, British Association of Social Workers
- Vicky Johnston, Chair, Chartered Physiotherapists Working with Older People
- Carley King, Professional Adviser, Chartered Society of Physiotherapy
- Mark Taylor, Chief Officer, North Norfolk Clinical Commissioning Group
- Andy Tilden, Director, Sector Development – Skills, Skills for Care
- Dr Jonathan Treml, Consultant Geriatrician, Queen Elizabeth Hospital, Birmingham, Associate Director/Clinical Lead of Falls Workstream, Falls and Fragility Fracture Audit Programme, and Co-Chair, British Geriatrics Society Falls and Bone Health Section on behalf of members of the British Geriatrics Society and Royal College of Physicians
- Catherine Trustram-Eve, British Association of Nutritional Therapies
- Julie Windsor, Patient Safety Lead for Older People and Falls, NHS England

4. External Peer Reviewers

- Dr Claire Ballinger FCOT, PhD, MSc, DipCOT, Senior Qualitative Methodologist, RDS South Central and Principal Research Fellow – PPI, CLAHRC Wessex

- Professor Avril Drummond FCOT, PhD, MSc, DipCOT, Professor of Healthcare Research, Director of Research, School of Health Sciences, University of Nottingham

- Associate Professor Alison Pighills PhD, MSc, DipCOT, Health Practitioner Research Capacity, Queensland Health/James Cook University, Queensland, Australia

5. Co-opted critical appraisers

- Susan Dewar BSc (Hons), Occupational Therapist, Hospital Discharge Team, West Dunbartonshire CHCP, Glasgow, and COTSS-Older People Falls Clinical Forum: Member

- Fiona Jones BSc Hons, Occupational Therapist, Community Integrated Intermediate Care Services, Bettws, Wales, and COTSS-Older People Falls Clinical Forum: Member

- Sheila Morris MSc, Occupational Therapist and Community Lead for Falls Prevention for NHS Scotland Highland, UK, and COTSS-Older People Falls Clinical Forum: Member

- Rachel Russell BSc Hons, MSc, Occupational Therapist, PhD candidate, School of the Built Environment, University of Salford, and COTSS-Older People Falls Clinical Forum: Member

- Mandy Sainty MSc, DipCOT, Research and Development Manager, College of Occupational Therapists

- Laura Stuart MSc, PGCert, BSc (Hons), Frailty Lead, UCL Partners, London, and COTSS-Older People Falls Clinical Forum: Member

- Karin Tancock PGDip, DipCOT, Professional Affairs Officer for Older People and Long Term Conditions, College of Occupational Therapists

- Dr Elizabeth White PhD, Head of Research and Development, College of Occupational Therapists

6. End users

The views of those members of the British Association of Occupational Therapists who commented on the scope and the draft guideline during the consultation periods were much appreciated.

Respondents included members of a number of the College of Occupational Therapists Specialist Sections: HIV, Oncology and Palliative Care; Housing; Neurological Practice; Older People; and Trauma and Orthopaedics.

7. The guideline development group would additionally like to thank the following:

- The College of Occupational Therapists' Library Service

- The College of Occupational Therapists' Practice Publications Group and supporting officers Julia Roberts, Quality Programme Manager and Tessa Woodfine, Publications Manager

Appendix 3: Conflicts of interest declarations

Declarations were made, in line with the conflict of interest procedures (see Section 4.6), as follows:

- All members of the core GDG membership were members of the COTSS-Older People.

- The co-opted editorial lead was an officer of the College of Occupational Therapists.

- Three of the co-opted critical appraisers were officers of the College of Occupational Therapists.

- Five of the co-opted critical appraisers were members of the COTSS-Older People Falls Clinical Forum.

- External peer reviewers declared authorship of one or more publications included in the guideline, and their status as researchers in falls.

- Guideline group members, external peer reviewers and stakeholders identified their membership of professional organisations or specialist falls-related forums.

- Stakeholder declarations included involvement in falls prevention working parties and forums, and research activities, within their work and organisational capacity.

Declarations were related to the expertise of the individuals who, through their professional interests, were members of specialist forums or organisations, or involved in falls prevention and management through their clinical, educational or research activities.

The peer reviewers, by the nature of their expertise, were authors of research used to support recommendations; as the views and opinions of three experts were obtained, this meant there was no undue bias.

Officers of the College of Occupational Therapists were involved in critical appraisal activities, but all evidence was appraised by two individuals and allocations ensured that these officers were paired with an appraiser from outside the College of Occupational Therapists.

No commercial or financial interests were declared.

Adherence to the College of Occupational Therapists' conflicts of interest policy, the nature and management of the above declarations, and the robust guideline development methodology mean that the potential for any bias has been taken into account.

Appendix 4: Service user consultation

Consultation took place on the draft guideline recommendations as outlined in Section 4.3. Feedback from phases 1 and 2 of the draft guideline consultation is provided below.

1. Do you think the explanation of what occupational therapy is and how occupational therapists promote independence is clear enough?

"It is very 'OT jargon' – accepting that this guideline is for OTs that is OK, BUT in the scoping document you did say that this guideline would be useful for others, including commissioners, so the definition needs to be simpler."

"Absolutely clear. The guidelines explain this well in easy to understand language."

"Yes, I think it is explained well."

2. Do you think the title is right, given that not all falls can be prevented?

"Yes, it is clear and unambiguous."

"No – the title should just be 'Falls: the role of occupational therapy in the management of falls in adults' as to use the word 'prevention' implies all falls could have been prevented."

With respect to the guideline title, the service user perspective was respected, but the use of the term "prevention" was retained in the guideline title for consultation. This is to reflect that the overarching objectives of occupational therapy include both prevention and management of falls, to be congruent with the national guideline focus, and to maximise the guideline's inclusion in the results of future falls topic literature searches.

3. Do you think the recommendations are easy to understand?

"Not all of them."

"Yes, the recommendations give a structure for therapists to work towards whilst allowing for changes based on clinical judgement to tailor interventions to a person-centred model."

"Could do with a few less words."

"Something could be added about outside activities."

4. Do you think these recommendations will help patients understand how they can reduce their risk of falling?

"Yes, if they want to listen!"

"Yes but only for those who do not have dementia or a loss of understanding."

"Hopefully. I think these recommendations will need to be published widely so people are aware of this type of service, most of the general public may not know this service exists."

"More home assessments are needed."

5. Do you think the word "safe" should be included?

"No – the problem with 'safe' is it can restrict activity so you 'stay safe' – nothing can ever be totally safe. It is about minimising risk."

Use of the word "safe" in the third recommendation category heading was an acceptable context.

6. Is the word "purposeful" useful?

"No – there are times when what you are doing or what you want to do does not necessarily have a purpose to it, i.e. 'purposeful' implies there should be a useful outcome."

7. Do the outcomes make sense?

"Yes."

"Yes. I really like how the outcomes focus on individuals and their own perception of falls and the impact this has on their daily lives, and also encourages the belief that positive changes are possible."

The service users' views were influential and insightful. All points raised were reviewed and, as a consequence, a number of amendments were made to both the pre-consultation draft and the final guideline document.

Appendix 5: Literature search strategy

Table A1: Search terms and strings

1	2	3	4	5	6
Falls and related terms	Psychological factors	Outcomes	Interventions	Occupational therapy and related terms	Occupational therapy
fall* OR recurrent fall* OR frequency of fall* OR context of fall* OR characteristic* of fall* OR accident* fall* OR mechan* fall* OR non-mechan* fall* OR trip* OR slip* OR drop attack OR drop-attack OR collapse OR syncope OR faint OR fragil* frac*	anxi* OR fear* OR confide* OR lifestyle limit* OR pyscho* OR motivat* OR perce* OR distress OR behaviour OR behaviour OR self eff* OR auton* OR dignity OR embarrass* OR wellbeing OR well-being	confiden* OR economic OR social OR behav* OR psycho* OR physical OR outcome measure OR independ* OR function* indep* OR identification* of hazard* OR environment* redesign OR lifestyle redesign OR prevent* OR rate of frac* OR inciden* of frac* OR inciden* of fall* OR rate of fall* OR management of fall* OR motivat* OR complian* OR coping or aware* OR quality of life OR positiv* risk taking OR medic* concord* OR medication manag* OR safety OR wellbeing OR well-being OR self care OR self-care OR personal care OR productiv* OR human cost* OR financ* cost*	assessment OR outcome measure OR intervention OR multifactorial assessment OR multifactorial intervention OR function OR goal setting OR problem solving OR seat* OR postur* propriocept* OR spatial OR spatial percept* OR discharge plan* OR manual hand* OR assistive tech* OR rehabilitat* OR cop* strat* OR contingen* plan* OR home hazard* reduc* OR hazard or home* OR environment* OR awareness OR moving OR handling OR neglect OR inattention OR attention OR equipment OR aids OR tele* OR virtual OR concentrat* OR modif* OR reasoning OR	lifestyle modif* OR daily liv* skil* OR daily liv* OR fall* prevention OR fall* program* or OR fall* management OR education OR self care OR self-care OR personal care OR self management OR rehabilit* OR sensory OR compensat* OR judgement OR insight OR in-sight	occupational therap* OR therap* OR rehab* OR reable* OR enable* OR multidis* OR multi-dis* OR unidiscip* OR undiscip* OR activit* OR occupat* OR life skill*	Occupational therap*

Table A2: Database search strategy

A title/abstract/descriptor search was undertaken. Each string combination (Table A1), dependent on the search database, was therefore automatically ended or preceded with the relevant term:

- Ovid platform search strings were followed by *.ti.* (title search), *.ab.* (abstract search) or *.de.* (descriptor search).
- EBSCO platform search strings were preceded by *TI* (title search), *AB* (abstract search) or *SU* (subject search).

The following table shows EBSCO (Medline, CINAHL) and Ovid (AMED, HMIC, PsycINFO, Social Policy and Practice) platform searches covering 1 January 2003 to search date in 2013:

Platform, search type and date	Search no.	Search strings (columns in Table A1)	Medline	CINAHL	AMED	HMIC	PsycINFO	Social Policy	Subtotal
Title search (EBSCO and Ovid search date 17.09.13)	S1	1 AND 2 AND 5	70	55	13	0	27	7	172
	S2	1 AND 3 AND 5	211	197	32	11	67	9	527
	S3	1 AND 4 AND 5	292	223	60	11	68	9	663
Total									**1362**
Title search (EBSCO search date 18.09.13, Ovid search date 17.09.13)	S4	1 AND 2 AND 6	9	14	0	0	1	0	24
	S5	1 AND 3 AND 6	20	38	6	1	5	1	71
	S6	1 AND 4 AND 6	28	43	7	1	5	1	85
Total									**180**
Abstract search (EBSCO and Ovid search date 18.09.13)	S7	1 AND 2 AND 6	54	53	27	7	26	8	175
	S8	1 AND 3 AND 6	135	107	49	19	71	24	405
	S9	1 AND 4 AND 6	85	115	49	16	68	22	355
Total									**935**

Platform, search type and date	Search no.	Search strings (columns in Table A1)	Medline	CINAHL	AMED	HMIC	PsycINFO	Social Policy	Subtotal
Descriptor search (EBSCO and Ovid search date 19.09.13)	S10	1 AND 2 AND 6	54	51	0	1	1	1	108
	S11	1 AND 3 AND 6	55	153	0	4	2	4	218
	S12	1 AND 4 AND 6	49	162	0	1	6	3	221
Total									547
Total search results									3024

Table A3: Specialist searches

Search description (no date range set, except OTDBASE 01.01.03–23.09.13)	Search date	Results
OTseeker: all fields search – 'fall*'	27.09.13	259
OTsearch: title field search – 'fall*'	27.09.13	61
OTDBASE: title field search for four terms – 'fall', 'falls', 'falling', 'fallen'	27.09.13	45
Cochrane Library: title, abstract and descriptor fields search – 'fall*' and 'occupational'	27.09.13	4
College of Occupational Therapists Thesis Collection: all fields search – 'fall*'	27.09.13	5
NHS Economic Evaluation Database (EED): title search – 'falls', all fields search – 'occupational therapy'	27.09.13	24
Total		398

Appendix 6: Evidence-based review tables

Source	Design and participants	Intervention	Outcomes	Results	Quality and comment
Ballinger et al (2006)	Qualitative study Aim: to investigate the perspectives of the older participants in a community group falls prevention programme in Australia and to explore their views about the most and least useful aspects of the programme, using methods derived from a grounded theory approach Participants were already members of a group attending a *Stepping On* falls prevention programme 11 participants Male: female ratio = 2:9 Age 69 to 91 years (median age of 76) Australia.	Intervention: 2-hour sessions in a community group setting once a week for 7 weeks Session: 1. Sharing fall experiences; strength and balance exercises 2. Exploring the barriers and benefits of exercise; mobilising safely 3. Home hazards 4. Community safety and footwear 5. Vision and falls 6. Medication management; mobility mastery experiences 7. Review and planning ahead Control: Two social visits from an occupational therapy student.	Semi structured interviews Interview schedule comprised 11 questions and was developed in conjunction with expert occupational therapists involved in falls prevention initiatives The interviews took place 3 months after the programme and all except the telephone interview were carried out in the participants' own homes. Interviews lasted 30–60 minutes.	4 themes identified: Identity: understanding of self in context of falls-prevention programme Salience of interventions: mostly good recall of programme but series of exercises appeared the most important single intervention. Less useful or relevant aspects referred to by some participants were medication, home hazards and, for men, the discussion about footwear Social experience: experience of being part of a friendly group reported as one of the most enjoyable aspects of the programme Consequences of participation: the programme fulfilled a variety of different needs and the outcomes that the participants identified were not always those that might have been predicted or expected An increase in confidence was the major psychological benefit described by participants Highlighted that perceived outcomes are connected to intrinsic values of independence and wellbeing.	Grade C – Low Comments: • Potential impact of previous contact with researcher as this study was part of a larger RCT.

Source	Design and participants	Intervention	Outcomes	Results	Quality and comment
Boltz et al (2013)	Mixed methods Aim: to describe fear of falling among older adults in acute care settings and consider the relationship between fear of falling and patient demographic and health characteristics, as well as physical function during the hospital stay Recruited from two medical or medical/surgical units Community-residing Age ≥ 70 years Exclusions: Cognitive score < 24 or less than 6 months life expectancy 41 participants Male: female ratio = 17:24 Mean age 81.7 years Semi-structured interviews between 48 and 96 hours after admission United States of America.	A number of quantitative measures were used to collect data A semi-structured interview guide, developed by the researchers, was used to explore perceptions around mobility and physical activity as well as fear of falling Participants were asked to describe facilitators and barriers to mobility and physical activity, if they were afraid of falling, and their views on fall prevention measures while hospitalised.	Socio-demographic and health information was extracted from the medical record Information was also collected by trained data collectors within 24 hours of admission: • Cognitive status (Folstein mini-mental status examination MMSE) • Affective status (Yale Depression Scale) • Fear of falling (single-item question asking 'how fearful of falling' with self-rating on scale of 0 to 4, with 4 being the most fear) • Activities of daily living status (Barthel Scale) • Gait and balance (Tinetti Performance Oriented Mobility assessment) An evaluation of functional performance was conducted on the day of discharge.	Key points: • Fear of falling linked with depression • Environment and lack of time by staff impact on restriction • Perceptions of need to stay in bed to avoid falls 28 (68.3%) participants described fear of falling (score of 2 or more on the single-item question). Those who described themselves as depressed were more likely to describe fear of falling (r=0.47 (correlation); p=0.002) The following broad themes were identified from the interview: • I'm here because I'm sick • Knowing who to count on • It's not safe to move here • It needs to work for what I want and need • Activity restriction (e.g. 'keeping still') versus self-direction (e.g. 'use your common sense') emerged as the predominant responses to the fear of falling across the theme Fear of falling in older people admitted to hospital results in activity restriction Participants described the hospital environment and the lack of age-adapted furniture and bathing/toileting facilities, appropriate bed heights, accessible mobility devices and safe walking areas Potential for fear of falling to negatively influence mobility, physical activity and functional performance in hospitalised older adults.	Grade C – Low Comments: • Sample size of 41 provided limited power for analysis for quantitative measures • All potential confounding variables not identified • There was no follow-up of participants post-discharge.

Source	Design and participants	Intervention	Outcomes	Results	Quality and comment
Campbell et al (2005) [Cross reference with La Grow et al 2006]	Randomised controlled trial Aim: to assess the efficacy and cost-effectiveness of a home safety programme and a home exercise programme to reduce falls and injuries in older people with low vision • Aged ≥ 75 years • Community dwelling • Poor vision • Mobile in own home • Not currently receiving physiotherapy 391 participants randomised to 4 groups: Home Safety Assessment and Modification 100 participants Male: female ratio = 34:66 Exercise Programme 97 participants Male: female ratio = 25:72 Home Safety Assessment and Exercise Programme 98 participants Male: female ratio = 36:62 Social visits 96 participants Male: female ratio = 29:67 Mean age 83.6 years New Zealand.	Home Safety Programme: Occupational therapy home visit (Westmead Home Safety Assessment); discuss and agree interventions and hazard reduction. Follow-up visit if required Telephone interview at 6 months to determine if recommendations for home modifications and behaviour change carried out, partially carried out or not carried out Exercise Programme: One year Otago programme modified for visual impairment and prescribed by physiotherapist, plus Vitamin D supplement Home safety and exercise programmes (as above) Social visits: Two one hour visits by research staff during first 6 months of the trial to those not randomised to other groups.	Falls: • Number • Injuries sustained • Monitored for one year Costs: Of implementing the home safety programme using the social visit group as comparator.	Participants who had occupational therapy safety programme had 41% fewer falls when compared to those who did not receive the programme (incidence rate ratio 0.59; 95% CI [0.42, 0.83]) Participants receiving the exercise programme had 15% fewer falls compared to those who did not receive the programme. Adherence was an issue for the exercise programme as stricter adherence was associated with fewer falls Demonstrated that the home safety programme, delivered by occupational therapists, was a more effective intervention in decreasing falls for those who are visually impaired The home safety programme cost £234 per fall prevented (2004 prices). It was more cost-effective in this group than the exercise programme The effectiveness of an occupational therapy home visit with agreed home and behaviour modifications appeared to result in significantly fewer falls both within and away from the home environment. This suggested an increased awareness of falls-reduction strategies within the home could generalise to the wider environment.	Grade A – High Comments: • Participants were recruited via Low Vision Clinics and Royal New Zealand Foundation for the Blind due to their visual impairment, not their ability to complete an exercise programme • Duration of visual impairment varied considerably among participants • Hard to extrapolate exactly where the effect of the intervention lies as within the home safety programme there were also fewer falls away from the home environment.

Source	Design and participants	Intervention	Outcomes	Results	Quality and comment
Clemson et al (2004)	Randomised controlled trial Aim: to test whether *Stepping On*, a multifaceted community-based programme using a small-group learning environment, is effective in reducing falls in at-risk people living at home 310 community dwelling older people Inclusions: • Age ≥ 70 years • Fallen in the previous 12 months or • Concerned about falling Exclusions: • Cognitive problems • Homebound/unable to independently leave home Intervention Group of 157 participants Male: female ratio = 40:117 Mean age 78.31 years 147 completed trial Control Group of 153 participants Male: female ratio = 40:113 Mean age 78.47 years 130 completed trial Australia.	Intervention Group: *Stepping On programme* aimed to improve fall self-efficacy, encourage behavioural change, and reduce falls. A variety of learning strategies were used: raising awareness; targeting behaviours that have the most effect on reducing risk and reinforcing their application to the individual's home and community setting; specific techniques such as storytelling, mastery experiences, and the group process as a learning environment Occupational therapist facilitated, two-hour sessions weekly for 7 weeks, average of 12 participants per group, follow-up occupational therapy home visit Control Group: Up to two social visits from an occupational therapy student instructed not to discuss falls or falls prevention with the subjects.	Primary outcome: • Number of falls Evaluation from baseline up to 14 months post-randomisation using a self-report falls schedule Baseline: • Demographics • Fall and health history • Get Up and Go Test (mobility and balance) • Rhomberg test (balance) Secondary outcomes: • Modified Falls Efficacy Scale (MFES) • Health survey SF-36® • Physical Activity Scale for the Elderly • Mobility Efficacy Score (MES) Additional measure at follow-up: • Falls Behavioural Scale (FaB).	The *Stepping On Programme* was effective in reducing falls, especially in men Primary outcome (number of falls): subgroup analyses found significant effects in older participants, men, those with intermediate levels of functional mobility and balance, those with previous falls. Statistically significant interaction was only for gender (p=0.003) Secondary outcomes: intervention group participants maintained confidence in ability to avoid a fall during a variety of functional daily living tasks over the follow-up period. A decrease in confidence was experienced by control group (MES, p=0.042) No difference detected in self-efficacy for more home-based daily living activities (MFES). More protective behavioural practices were used by intervention group than control subjects (FaB, p=0.024) Intervention group experienced a 31% reduction in falls (relative risk 0.69, 95% CI [0.50, 0.96]; p=0.025) – a clinically meaningful result demonstrating the *Stepping On programme* was effective for older people living in the community 70% (n=80) of programme participants adhered to at least 50% of the home visit recommendations Study findings provided some evidence that cognitive-behavioural learning in a small group environment could reduce falls.	Grade A – High Comments: • Participants were not housebound so less frail than those more often seen at home due to falls • Difference in contact time between intervention and control group may have caused bias.

Source	Design and participants	Intervention	Outcomes	Results	Quality and comment
Clemson et al (2008)	Systematic review and meta-analysis Aim: to determine the efficacy of environmental interventions in falls prevention and increase the precision of results by pooling eligible studies Inclusions: • RCTs • Living in the community • Aged ≥ 65 years • Home environment intervention as single intervention 388 abstracts screened 6 trials met inclusion criteria Pooled analysis of the six trials (3,298 participants) Mean age of participants 79.6 years Australia (3 trials), New Zealand, Germany and France.	The analysis included single component trials i.e. where environment intervention only completed or where the environment component could be isolated Studies that included an environmental intervention as a component of a multifaceted intervention were not included.	Primary outcome: rate of falls expressed as relative risk Interventions were rated according to the level of professional training of the interventionist and the intensity of the intervention Comprehensive meta-analysis software was used to generate pooled estimates of effect sizes.	Modest but significant reduction in falls: 21% reduction in falls risk across all studies included (relative risk 0.79; 95% CI [0.65, 0.97]) Sub-analysis of high-risk populations: history of falls in previous 12 months, hospitalised due to fall, functional decline and visual impairment (n=570 across 4 trials) identified clinically significant reduction of falls 39% reduction of falls (relative risk 0.61; 95% CI [0.47, 0.79]) across high-risk populations (an absolute risk difference of 26% for a number needed to treat four people) Some evidence to suggest that interventions when completed by occupational therapist at higher intensity were more effective Results identified that the highest effects in terms of reducing falls were associated with interventions targeted to high-risk groups.	Grade A – High Comments: • Limited ability to complete sub-analysis therefore limiting richness of information i.e. information on injuries, age, gender, co-morbidities etc • Small number of high-quality published papers where the environment is single component or can be isolated from multifactorial study.

Source	Design and participants	Intervention	Outcomes	Results	Quality and comment
Clemson et al (2010) [Cross reference with Clemson et al 2012]	Randomised controlled trial Aim: to conduct a small scale investigation into the feasibility and efficacy of the novel LiFE intervention Recruited from Department of Veterans Affairs Home Front database and a General Medical Practice Community-residing Aged ≥ 70 years Two or more falls or an injurious fall in past year Individuals randomised to: Intervention group of 18 participants Male: female ratio = 9:9 Mean age 81 years Control group of 16 participants Male: female ratio = 9:7 Mean age 82 years Exclusions: moderate to severe cognitive problems, inability to ambulate independently, nursing home or hostel resident, unstable/terminal illness precluding planned exercises, neurological conditions with motor performance difficulties Australia.	LiFE involved teaching core underlying principles of balance and strength training, which were operationalised into four balance strategies and seven strength strategies; applied in individualised activities and incorporated into daily activities such as ironing, cleaning teeth The LiFE manual provided to participants outlined the programme in detail Intervention Group: LiFE taught in five home visits with two booster visits over a three-month period and two follow-up phone calls The focus was on choosing safe, contextually relevant activities and upgrading the activities over time Control Group: usual care.	Baseline assessment occurred prior to randomisation and was repeated at three and six months. Outcome measures included: • Rate of falls (falls calendar) • Physical capacity (balance and strength) • Health Status Survey (SF-36®) • Modified Falls Efficacy Scale (FES Scale), • Activities-Specific Balance Confidence Scale (ABC Scale) • Life Space Assessment (measures the geographical space used and travelled) Exercise adherence was monitored for six months by the treating therapist using weekly and monthly logs.	Completed follow up at 6 months: 17/18 intervention group, 12/16 control group After 6 months there were 12 falls in the intervention group and 35 in the control group 8 (44%) intervention and 9 (31%) control participants reported one or more falls 3 (17%) intervention and 6 (31%) control participants reported two or more falls The relative risk analysis demonstrated a significant reduction in falls (relative risk 0.23; 95% CI [0.07, 0.83]) There were significant improvements in the intervention group compared with the controls for dynamic balance and left knee strength in the first three months. Balance self-efficacy improved significantly in the intervention group at the end of six months. Falls self-efficacy was significantly improved in the intervention group at three months, a difference maintained at six months but not significantly different from controls at that time point No difference was noted in perceptions of health-related quality of life The Life Space Scale showed zero change for either group LiFE was feasible in terms of study design, and demonstrated effectiveness in reducing recurrent falls in this at-risk sample.	Grade B – Moderate Downgraded from Grade A due to limitations: • Caution is needed in interpreting results given this is a pilot study • Small sample of participants is under-powered • Unequal rate of dropout (25% controls compared with 6% from the intervention group) and thus potential for contamination if the controls sought other programmes • Single-blinded outcome assessment (assessors blinded).

Source	Design and participants	Intervention	Outcomes	Results	Quality and comment
Clemson et al (2012) *[Cross reference with Clemson et al 2010]*	Randomised controlled trial Aim: to determine if the integration of the LiFE approach is effective in reducing the rate of falls in older, high risk people living at home Recruited from Veteran Affairs Database and GP databases based in metropolitan Sydney ≥ 2 falls or 1 injurious fall in the last 6 months Exclusions: moderate to severe cognitive problems, inability to ambulate independently, neurological conditions severely influencing gait and mobility, nursing home or hostel resident, unstable or terminal illness affecting ability to do exercises 317 participants Age ≥ 70 years Male: female ratios are: LiFE group 48:59 Exercise group 48:57 Control group 47:58 Australia.	The 3 randomised parallel blocks were: 1) LiFE approach (n=107) Taught principals of balance and strength training and integrated selected activities into everyday routines Examples provided of dual tasking LiFE activities are ironing while standing on one leg; squatting to select an item from a low shelf rather than bending 2) Structured programme (n=105) Exercises for balance and lower limb completed 3 × weekly Blocks 1 and 2 received 5 × sessions with 2 booster visits and 2 telephone calls 3) Sham control group (n=105) Gentle exercise.	Assessments completed at baseline, 6 months and 12 months Primary outcomes: • Rate of falls over 12 months collected by self-report Secondary measures included: • Static and dynamic balance • Ankle, hip strength • Balance self-efficacy (ABC Scale) • Daily living activities functional limitation (Late Life Function Index, NHANES independence measure) • Life tasks participation (Late Life Disability Index) • Habitual physical exercise (Physical Activity Scale for the Elderly) • Health related quality of life (EQ-5D) • Energy expenditure (Paffenbarger physical activity index).	The overall incidence of falls in the LiFE group (1.66 per person years) was lower than that of the structured exercise (1.90) and control groups (2.28) respectively There was a significant 31% reduction in rate of falls with the LiFE group compared with the control programme (incidence rate ratio 0.69; 95% CI [0.48, 0.99], n=212) Comparing the structured programme to the control, there was no significant reduction in the fall rate Static balance on eight level hierarchy scale, ankle strength, function and participation was significantly better in the LiFE group compared with the other groups There was a significant and moderate improvement in dynamic balance in the LiFE and structured groups compared with the control group The LiFE programme offered an alternative to traditional exercise as a falls prevention intervention.	Grade A – High Comments: • The study had a lower sample size than preferred which could lead to a type 2 error • The control group received less contact time than both interventions, which could have caused a bias.

Source	Design and participants	Intervention	Outcomes	Results	Quality and comment
Costello and Edelstein (2008)	Systematic review Review of randomised controlled trials that investigated the effectiveness of fall prevention programmes for community-dwelling older adults Inclusions: • RCTs • Published between 1996 and 2007 • Age ≥ 60 years • Ambulatory with or without an assistive device • Community dwelling • Single or multifactorial interventions Eight databases searched Countries in which studies conducted not defined.	Studies were grouped according to the following types of intervention programmes: • Home hazard assessment with modification only (n=4) • Exercise and/or physical therapy only (n=10) • Programmes that offered multifactorial intervention (n=12).	Number of falls, number of fallers and rate of falls.	The inclusion criteria were met by 781 studies, 26 of which were included in the review The review determined the following with respect to interventions: • Multifactorial fall prevention programmes included in this review indicated that they were more effective when targeted for those older individuals with a previous fall history • A falls screening examination should include medication and vision assessment with appropriate health practitioner referral • Exercise alone is effective in reducing falls; it should include a comprehensive programme combining muscle strengthening, balance, and/or endurance training for a minimum of 12 weeks • Home hazard assessment with modifications may be beneficial in reducing falls, especially in a targeted group of individuals.	Grade B – Moderate Downgraded from Grade A due to limitations: • Heterogeneous nature of studies • Good critical analysis rather than stringent systematic review • Not possible to undertake meta-analysis • Large range of exclusion criteria in studies • Some of the variation in outcomes between individual studies and comprehensive reviews may be due to variations and inaccuracies in fall data collection.

Source	Design and participants	Intervention	Outcomes	Results	Quality and comment
Currin et al (2012)	Cohort study Aim: to identify the uptake of home modifications made by occupational therapists to reduce falls risks by older community dwellers and to identify the intrinsic and extrinsic factors that predict uptake of recommendations Recruited from concurrent randomised controlled trial Community dwelling Recent fall 80 participants Age > 60 years Male: female ratio 24:56 Australia.	Joint occupational therapist and physiotherapist home visit List of environmental recommendations generated by the occupational therapist following completion of the home visit At 6-month follow-up, an independent assessor not involved with the trial visited the clients at their homes and identified whether the recommendations were completed.	Falls Prevention Environmental Audit used to measure environment Number of recommendations implemented at 6-month follow-up.	63 follow-up visits made. 17 participants lost to follow-up 277 recommendations were made: 200 required participant to act; 77 completed by other agencies 106 recommendations were for bathroom and toilet, 39 for passageways 136 (49%) of recommendations completed by follow-up 50% of recommendations for rails in shower and toilet, non-slip bath mats, bed sticks and stair rails completed Participants less likely to implement over-toilet frames, shower chairs or altering floor surfaces including removing rugs • Adherence increased with increasing co-morbidities • Adherence improved when referred to outside agency • Adherence lower where participant had depression/psychological distress The full potential of an occupational therapy environmental audit recommendations will only be achieved if recommended modifications are actually implemented Adherence is a complex process and has multiple influences impacting on the outcome.	Grade C – Low Comments: • Recruitment bias potential as participants already active in RCT • Effect of advice given by occupational therapist during visit not considered or accounted for • All occupational therapy staff received same training pre-study but no account for differing skill sets/experience • No validity or reliability data given for home hazard assessment used • Most participants on low income, therefore unable to determine effect of income on uptake of recommendations.

Source	Design and participants	Intervention	Outcomes	Results	Quality and comment
de Groot and Fagerström al (2011)	Qualitative study Aim: to describe motivating factors and barriers for older adults to adhere to group exercise in the local community aiming to prevent falls Recruited from a previous exercise group study prompted by high dropout rate when exercise group moved from hospital to the community setting Older adults with equal representation of those with fear of falling and those with no fear of falling and variation in travelling distance to attend the group 10 participants Age 71–91 years Mean 83 years Male: female ratio = 5:5 Semi-structured individual interviews in participants own homes Norway.	Interview followed 9 themed areas: • Personal data • Question about previous study • Engagement in physical activity and exercise • Types of exercise • Regularity of exercise • Fear of falling and actual falls • Contact with health professionals • Distance to venue and economics burden of transport • Health status.	Theoretical framework was the motivation equation ascertaining motivation and barriers Identifies 4 main factors which are modifiable: • Perceived chance of success • Perceived importance of the goal • Perceived costs • Inclination to remain sedentary.	Factors which enhanced motivation to adhere to the recommended exercise were: • Perceived prospects of remaining independent • Maintaining current health status • Improving physical balance • Ability to walk Barriers included: • Reduced health status • Lack of motivation • Unpleasant experience in previous group exercise session • Environmental factors (transport, weather) Other relevant factors for adherence were the positive impact of social interaction from the group and the provision of adequate information by health professionals Older adults will be motivated in a variety of ways and by different factors. Identifying an individual's essential motivating factors and barriers is important.	Grade C – Low Comments: • Researcher from previous study recruited and interviewed participants which might have led to bias • Some participants contacted via letter, others by telephone • Limited selection of centres where previous study held programmes • Time from discontinuing a group exercise course to the interview varied which might have influenced participant recall.

Source	Design and participants	Intervention	Outcomes	Results	Quality and comment
Di Monaco et al (2008) *[Cross reference with Di Monaco et al 2012]*	Quasi-randomised controlled trial Aim: to assess the role of a post-discharge home visit by an occupational therapist in reducing the risk of falling in hip fracture women Recruited from consecutive patients admitted to a rehabilitation hospital in Turin because of hip fracture. • All women • Age ≥ 60 years • Sustained a fall-related hip fracture • Mini Mental State Examination score higher than 23 Alternate allocation to study and control groups Intervention Group of 58 participants Control Group of 61 participants Italy.	All participants received treatment as usual, a multi-professional intervention to prevent falls delivered 1–3 hours a day for 5 days a week, conducted by physiotherapists and occupational therapists Included occupational therapist assessing (form information) any home-hazards of falling based on a standard checklist and based on patient's behaviour during activities of daily living Intervention Group: additionally received a home visit by an occupational therapist at a median point of 20 days post-discharge. Involved assessment of environmental hazards, behaviours in activities of daily living, use of assistive devices and suggested targeted modifications to prevent falls (mean time of 60 minutes).	Occurrence of falls All women were asked to record all falls occurring post-discharge and report them at a home visit by an occupational therapist scheduled for approximately 6 months post-discharge During the visit the occupational therapist asked the women in detail about: • Falls occurrence post-discharge • Level of adherence to the advice given during the first home visit was checked for the women in the intervention group (with the percentage of advice followed by each woman recorded).	Intervention Group analysis (n=45 – nine lost eligibility after randomisation and four lost to follow up, mean age 79.9 years): 6 participants sustained a fall (9 falls in total) during 8970 days post-discharge Control Group analysis (n=50 – seven lost eligibility after randomisation and four lost to follow up, mean age 80.1 years): 13 participants sustained a fall (20 falls in total) during 9231 days post-discharge A significantly lower proportion of fallers was found in the intervention group (odds ratio 0.275; 95% CI [0.081, 0.937], p=0.039) after adjustments In the intervention group a mean of 3.9 items of advice were given to each of the 45 women, 44 of whom followed at least one. 36 of the women followed at least half of the advice given during the first home visit The risk of falling in a sample of elderly women following hip fracture (who followed the occupational therapists advice delivered during a home visit) was significantly reduced by a single home visit by an occupational therapist 20 days after discharge from a rehabilitation hospital.	Grade B – Moderate Downgraded from Grade A due to limitations: • 95/270 originally considered included, potential participants excluded for a variety of reasons • All participants received extensive in-patient falls prevention training and this may have impacted on subsequent falls when compared with other studies • Unclear how generalisable results are to a wider population of hip fracture patients (women only) • Bias possible as same staff assessed falls and conducted the home visits • Follow up period was modest at 6 months.

Source	Design and participants	Intervention	Outcomes	Results	Quality and comment
Di Monaco et al (2012) *[Cross reference with Di Monaco et al 2008]*	Cohort study Post-hoc analysis of a quasi-randomised controlled trial (Di Monaco et al 2008) Aim: to investigate the value of falls risk assessment performed before hospital discharge in predicting falls occurrence. Also assessed the role of adherence to targeted recommendations given during the hospital stay in affecting the falls risk • Rehabilitation hospital • All women • Age ≥ 60 years • Sustained a fall-related hip fracture • Mini Mental State Examination score higher than 23 Alternate allocation to study and control groups Intervention Group of 58 participants Control Group of 61 participants Italy.	All participants received treatment as usual, a multi-professional intervention to prevent falls delivered 1–3 hours a day for 5 days a week, conducted by physiotherapists and occupational therapists Included occupational therapist assessing (form information) any home-hazards of falling based on a standard checklist and based on patient's behaviour during activities of daily living Intervention Group: additionally received a home visit by an occupational therapist at a median point of 20 days post-discharge. Involved assessment of environmental hazards, behaviours in activities of daily living, use of assistive devices and suggested targeted modifications to prevent falls (mean time of 60 minutes).	Occurrence of falls All women were asked to record all falls occurring post-discharge and report them at a home visit by an occupational therapist scheduled for approximately 6 months post-discharge. During the visit the occupational therapist asked the women in detail about: • Falls occurrence post-discharge • Level of adherence to the advice given during the first home visit was checked for the women in the intervention group (with the percentage of advice followed by each woman recorded) The post-hoc analysis included an assessment of the difference in the number of uncorrected risk factors in fallers and non-fallers.	The quasi-RCT (Di Monaco 2008) showed a significant reduction in the proportion of fallers who received a single visit by an occupational therapist post-discharge from hospital 95 women included in the analysis. Mean age 80 years In the post-hoc analysis 20% (19/95) of women in the study fell in the 6-month follow-up period. This was lower than other studies where the rate of falls post-hip fracture was 53% – a suggestion was made that this may have been due to the fact all women in the trial received a multidisciplinary falls intervention whilst in hospital Fall occurrence was significantly predicted by uncorrected environmental and behavioural factors, with a 4.58 odds ratio for the women in the high risk group (presence of 2 or more uncorrected risk factors) A significant reduction in falls risk was associated with high adherence to targeted recommendations, suggesting that adherence can have a key role in falls prevention and therefore strategies to enhance this are important.	Grade C – Low Comments: • Original study sample not representative of all hip fracture patients and thus limits the generalisability of the findings • Follow-up was only for 6 months • Time to first fall not recorded • Reporting of falls relied on participant recall at 6 months therefore under-reporting may have occurred.

Source	Design and participants	Intervention	Outcomes	Results	Quality and comment
Gillespie et al (2012)	Review (Cochrane) Aim: to establish which fall prevention interventions are effective for older people living in the community Inclusions: • Age ≥ 60 years • Living in the community, either at home or in places of residence that did not provide residential health-related care or rehabilitative services • Randomised controlled trials and quasi-randomised trials Included trials were from 21 countries.	Assessed the effects of interventions designed to reduce the incidence of falls in older people living in the community Data assessed and extracted from 159 trials with 79,193 participants.	Primary outcomes: • Rate of falls • Number of fallers Secondary outcomes: • Number of participants sustaining fall-related fractures • Adverse effects of the interventions • Economic outcomes.	Results of relevance to guideline: • Group and home-based exercise programmes, including Tai Chi, reduce rate of falls. Exercise intervention overall significantly reduced the risk of sustaining a fracture related to a fall • The rate of falls, but not the risk of falling, was reduced by the provision of multifactorial assessment and intervention programmes • Overall, Vitamin D supplementation did not appear to reduce falls or risk of falls. There may be some benefit for those with lower Vitamin D levels before treatment • Intervention to treat vision problems could lead to an increase in the rate and risk of falls – this may be related to previous activity levels • No evidence was found for cognitive behavioural interventions on the rate of falls Home safety assessment and modification interventions: • Effective in reducing rate of falls from analysis of 6 trials with 4208 participants (rate ratio 0.81; 95% CI [0.68, 0.97]) • Effective in reducing risk of falling from analysis of 7 trials with 4051 participants (rate ratio 0.88; 95% CI [0.80 to 0.96]) • Were more effective in people at higher risk of falling, including those with severe visual impairment The review also identified that home safety interventions appear to be more effective when delivered by an occupational therapist.	Grade A – High Comments: • Many trials specifically excluded older people with cognitive impairment so the results of this review may not be applicable to these people at risk • People with Parkinson's and those who were post-stroke were excluded from this review.

Source	Design and participants	Intervention	Outcomes	Results	Quality and comment
Gopaul and Connelly (2012)	Serial case studies: mixed methods Aim: investigated how knowledge of one's own fall risk influenced self-reported behaviours and beliefs about falls and fall prevention in the home by older adults Volunteers recruited from the retired community Fallen once in their home within the past 12 months, and did not require medical attention for injury from the fall Exclusions: uncontrolled medical conditions, scored lower than 17/22 on a Mini Mental State Examination 8 participants Male: female ratio = 6:2 Mean age 78.8 years Qualitative interviews occurring before and after quantitative measures to gather pre- and post-intervention data Canada.	Intervention provided: • An individualised report of participants' scores for three questionnaires and three fall-related outcome measures • Personalised booklet comprised of a home safety checklist for fall prevention and photographs of rooms in their own homes with environmental hazards circled and identified as a fall risk Interviews included discussion about fall and completion of outcome measures and questionnaires. Post intervention explored if there was an effect on falls and fall prevention beliefs and behaviours after receiving their individual estimate of fall risk.	Balance outcome measures: • Biodex Balance System SDTM • Berg Balance Scale • Timed Up and Go Questionnaires: • Falls Behavioural Scale for the Older Person (FaB) • Falls Efficacy Scale (FES) • Activities-specific Balance Confidence (ABC) Scale.	Emerging themes about perception of falls and risk from interviews: • Process of being aware • Having concern and being careful • Accepting • 'Action'/Behaviour related to fall prevention Majority of participants made home safety changes (n=7) and protective behaviours increased (n=6 as self-reported) Some inconsistency in findings between fall risk and expressed beliefs; expression of being 'fine' In addition to the many physical factors related to falls the results suggested that individual beliefs and behaviour contributed to this complex health issue for older adults A recurring barrier identified with respect to the uptake of fall prevention was admitting to being susceptible to falling and the associated consequences, noted as not wanting to 'do' fall prevention.	Grade D – Very Low Comments: • Excluded unstable health conditions or those using a wheelchair or scooter for mobility • Small sample size of older adults who fell in their homes, and not those who fell outside, could limit generalisability • Some indirectness of the findings • Residents had different levels of support at home, greater proportion of females and other baseline variables.

Source	Design and participants	Intervention	Outcomes	Results	Quality and comment
Haines et al (2004) *[Cross reference with Haines et al 2006]*	Randomised controlled trial Aim: to assess the effectiveness of a targeted, multiple intervention falls prevention programme in reducing falls and injuries related to falls in a sub-acute hospital Recruitment from consecutive admission to three wards (metropolitan sub-acute hospital setting) over 10-month period Intervention group of 310 participants Male: female ratio = 101:209 Control group of 316 participants Male: female ratio = 105:211 Age range 38 to 99 years (Mean age 80 years) Australia.	Intervention group: • Falls risk alert card targeted at family members/care givers • Exercise programme of 3 × 45 minute tailored sessions per week conducted by a research physiotherapist • Education programme of twice weekly individual sessions (up to 30 minutes) conducted by a research occupational therapist at participant's bedside. Education manual. Programme curriculum was covered over 4 sessions (2 weeks) and could be repeated if required • Hip Protectors Control group: Usual care of medical assessments, 1 hour sessions of physiotherapy and occupational therapy each weekday, plus 24 hour nursing and other allied services.	Primary outcomes on an intention to treat basis were analysed • Cumulative incidence of falls over time • Compared the incidence of falls with injuries between groups • Proportion of participants who experienced one or more falls during their hospital stay.	Intervention group had 30% fewer falls than the control group (149 versus 105). This was most obvious after 45 days of intervention when fall rate in control group marginally increased and rate in intervention group suddenly reduced (p=0.004) Intervention group had a lower proportion of participants who experienced one or more falls (71 versus 54) 35 participants fell once in the intervention group compared to 49 in the control group The intervention group had only 6 participants who fell four or more times compared to 9 in the control group The incidence of falls with injuries was 28% lower in the intervention group Results indicated that the targeted prevention programme including multiple interventions could reduce the incidence rates of falls in the sub-acute setting.	Grade B – High Downgraded from Grade A due to limitations: • No consideration of which of the multi-targeted interventions had a more effective outcome • Staff used clinical judgement to determine need/appropriateness of each intervention • Recommendations for each participant were different and they did not all undergo exactly the same interventions • Variable of cognitive state and impact on intervention application • Not completed blinded – may have influenced recording of incidence of falls or altered elements of 'usual care'.

Source	Design and participants	Intervention	Outcomes	Results	Quality and comment
Haines et al (2006) [Cross reference with Haines et al 2004]	Subgroup analysis of randomised controlled trial Aim: to evaluate the effectiveness of a patient education programme for preventing falls in the sub-acute hospital setting (sub-analysis of a larger RCT of a multiple intervention programme) 226 participants (subgroups of RCT with 626 participants) Recruitment via referrals to the education group by the hospital occupational therapist Eligibility: at high risk of falls and potential to benefit Exclusions: severe communication or learning difficulty Intervention group of 115 participants. Male: female ratio = 35:80 Mean age 83 years Control group of 111 participants. Male: female ratio = 40:71 Mean age 82 years Australia.	Education programme: 1:1 sessions including falls risk factor screen, consequences of falls, profile of falls within the inpatient unit, mechanisms of falls, practical steps which participants could take to avoid falls, participant quiz, goal setting and review Number of sessions varied ranging from 2–5 (average 4) Sessions varied in length from 15–35 minutes Sessions followed the same format, covering the same content Education delivered by a research occupational therapist.	Primary outcome: • Number of falls per 1000 patient days • Number of fallers Data gathered via hospital reporting procedures and hospital medical records Secondary outcome: patient knowledge and experience for which a questionnaire was developed.	All participants recommended for education: falls rate was 26 per 1000 patient days; fallers were 16% (relative risk 1.21) Participants receiving education only: falls rate was 4 per 1000 patient days; fallers were 3% (relative risk 2.19) Any participant recommended for education with Mini Mental State Examination (MMSE) > 23/30 = 11 falls per 1000 patient days; fallers were 11% (relative risk 1.59) Any participant recommended for education intervention with MMSE < 23/30 = 15 falls per 1000 patient days; fallers were 23% (relative risk 1.00) Intervention group had significantly lower incidence of falls than control in terms of falls per 1000 patient days but number of fallers was not significant Education evaluated at the end of sessions and not over time so difficult to determine the sustainability of the education in terms of falls reduction i.e. once the person is at home will they continue to modify their behaviour Difficult to conclude that one to one education alone reduces falls but a multifactorial intervention which includes education was effective at reducing falls.	Grade C – Low Comments: • Hospital staff and participants not blinded to study • Referral relied on judgment of hospital occupational therapist • Participants exposed to up to 3 other interventions • Participants exposed to information at different stages of rehabilitation and differing number or length of sessions • Poor completion rate (64/115) of questionnaires • Researcher delivered sessions and questionnaire may have introduced bias.

Source	Design and participants	Intervention	Outcomes	Results	Quality and comment
Hill et al (2009)	Randomised controlled trial

Aim: to evaluate the effectiveness of falls prevention education delivered to hospitalised older people via digital video disc (DVD) or written workbook on perceived falls risk, knowledge of, and motivation to engage in, falls prevention strategies

Recruitment via hospital wards and units

Age ≥ 60 years

Exclusions:
Mini Mental State Examination < 24/30, medically unstable, severe vision or hearing deficits

Phase 1 Quasi-experimental control group of 122 participants
Male: female ratio = 54:68

Phase 2 Randomised allocation to:

DVD group of 49 participants
Male: female ratio = 18:31

Workbook group of 51 participants
Male: female ratio = 25:26

Australia. | All participants received usual ward orientation and ad hoc falls prevention advice on admission

Intervention Groups:

Participants received the DVD (14 minutes in duration) or workbook education at their bedside for up to one hour

Both formats contained identical content (based on the Health Belief Model), which included information on the risk of falls, fall related harms and falls prevention strategies that could be undertaken within the hospital setting to reduce the risk of falling

Control Group:

Did not receive any specific falls prevention education from the investigators. | Custom-designed survey measuring perception of falls risk and harms and motivation to reduce general risk of falling on a five-point Likert scale of strongly agree to strongly disagree and knowledge of falls

Perceived risk of falling was assessed in both intervention groups prior to the education

The complete survey was administered immediately after the education

Comparisons were not made against the 'control' group for all aspects as the no-education control group was assessed on five knowledge survey items only. | A greater proportion of participants from the two intervention groups (combined) provided 'desired responses' for the 5 knowledge items compared to the control (p<0.001)

The two intervention groups were comparable prior to the education in self-perceived risk of falls (p=0.72)

Number of reported falls before study enrolment were comparable for the education groups (DVD, n=7; workbook, n=14; p=0.42) and control group (n=15; p=0.72)

Post-education there was no significant difference between the education groups in self-perceived falls risk (p=0.70) or knowledge of falls. There was a within group increase in the self-perceived risk of falls in the DVD group after the education (p=0.04); there was not a significant change within the workbook group

A higher proportion of participants in the DVD group were strongly motivated to prevent themselves from falling compared with the workbook group (60% versus 34%; p=0.04), and had greater confidence in their ability to do so (67% versus 45%; p=0.03)

The DVD education, when compared with a written workbook, had the potential to result in better update of information, influence perceptions and motivation with respect to falls prevention activities in the hospital setting. | Grade B – Moderate

Downgraded from Grade A due to limitations:

• Relatively small sample and no size calculation included
• Control group quasi-experimental and not randomised
• Bias as participants aware of education group
• Investigators conducting assessments aware of allocation group
• Not known if positive educational outcomes were followed by behaviour change, and whether associated with a reduction in falls in the hospital setting
• Unclear whether subjects retained the knowledge they gained. |

Source	Design and participants	Intervention	Outcomes	Results	Quality and comment
Johnston et al (2010)	Prospective, observational cohort study Aim: to describe the association between pre-discharge home assessment and falls in the first month post-discharge from a metropolitan rehabilitation hospital Consecutive admissions 342 participants Pre-discharge home visits for 223 participants. Median age 78 years Male: female ratio = 76:147 No home visit for 119 participants Median age 77 years Male: female ratio = 37:82 Exclusions: • Mini Mental State Examination < 24 • Significant psychiatric conditions • Admitted from, or had a planned discharge to a residential care facility • Unable to participate in telephone follow-up Australia.	Pre-discharge home visit versus no pre-discharge home visit On admission to the rehabilitation hospital, participants were classified into broad diagnostic groups All patients (whether participating in the study or not) were assessed by one of 17 occupational therapists working at the hospital The decision regarding provision of home assessment was made by the treating occupational therapist on clinical reasoning grounds.	Phase 1: Information gained from participants' medical record: • Falls Risk Assessment Scoring System (FRASS) • Functional performance (Functional Independence Measure [FIM™]) • Whether they had received an occupational therapy home assessment pre-discharge Phase 2: Prospective data following discharge: • Participants recorded any fall and associated details in a diary for a period of 1 month.	50 falls were recorded by 50 patients during the first month post-discharge (one fall per faller). 10.3% (23/223 patients) of the participants who received a home assessment reported a fall compared with 23.1% (27/119 patients) of those who did not. A pre-discharge home assessment was associated with a significantly decreased likelihood of falling during the first month post-discharge (odds ratio was 0.39; 95% CI [0.2, 0.75]; p=0.003) Not conducting a pre-discharge home assessment was associated with nearly three times the risk of falling in the month after discharge. However post-discharge fall risk of participants in the neurological group was not ameliorated by a home assessment Participants who received a home assessment had higher FRASS scores and lower FIM™ scores on both admission and discharge than those who did not Diagnosis, fall risk and functional independence scores indicated the participants for whom the protective effect of a home assessment was the strongest Occupational therapy home visit/assessments decreased risks of falls post-discharge.	Grade C – Low Comments: • Small sample size of subgroups • No details of clinical level of occupational therapists providing the treatment.

Source	Design and participants	Intervention	Outcomes	Results	Quality and comment
Kempen et al (2009)	Cross-sectional study Aim: to analyse univariate and multivariate associations between five socio-demographic, seven health-related and six psychosocial variables and levels of fear of falling and avoidance of activity in older persons who avoid activity due to fear of falling Local registry offices random sample 7,431 Community living people Age ≥ 70 years Sent a screening questionnaire, 4,376 responses Inclusion criteria: mild fear of falling and at least mild avoidance of activity due to fear of falling Exclusions: bed bound, wheelchair user, nursing home residents 540 participants Male: female ratio = 152:388 Netherlands.	Self-reported screening assessment and telephone interviews.	Fear of falling: Are you afraid of falling? Avoidance of activity: Do you avoid certain activities due to fear of falling? Socio demographic variables Health related variables: • Activities of daily living (Groningen Activity Restriction Scale) • Impaired vision and hearing • Perceived general health • Number of chronic conditions • Cognition (Telephone Interview for Cognitive Status) • Falls history Psychosocial variables: • General self-efficacy • Mastery scale • Social Support Scale • Hospital Anxiety and Depression Scale.	The study showed an interrelationship with socio demographics, health related and psychosocial variables in older people Female gender, limitations in activity of daily living and one or more falls in previous six months correlated independently with severe fear of falling Avoidance of activity in older people with severe levels of fear of falling may be particularly high in those of advanced age and with limitations in activities of daily living Old age, female gender, limitations in activities of daily living, impaired vision, poor perceived health, chronic morbidity, falls, low general self-efficacy, low mastery, loneliness, feelings of anxiety, and symptoms of depression were identified as univariate correlates of severe fear of falling and avoidance of activity May indicate concepts for developing interventions to reduce fear of falling and activity avoidance in old age.	Grade C – Low Comments: • Measures used were self-reported without the inclusion of performance-based measures • The sample only included people who reported to have a mild fear of falling and activity avoidance • Heterogeneous sample of people.

Source	Design and participants	Intervention	Outcomes	Results	Quality and comment
La Grow et al (2006) *[Cross reference with Campbell et al 2005]*	Randomised controlled trial Aim: to investigate whether the success of a home safety assessment and modification intervention in reducing falls resulted directly from modification of home hazards, from behavioural modifications or both • Aged ≥ 75 years • Community dwelling • Poor vision • Mobile in own home • Not currently receiving physiotherapy 391 participants were randomised to 4 groups: • Home Safety Assessment and Modification (100 participants) • Exercise Programme (97 participants) • Home Safety Assessment and Modification and Exercise Programme (98 participants) • Social visits (96 participants) New Zealand.	Home Safety Programme: Occupational therapy home visit (Westmead Home Safety Assessment); discuss and agree interventions and hazard reduction. Follow-up visit if required Telephone interview at 6 months to determine if recommendations for home modifications and behaviour change carried out, partially carried out or not carried out Exercise Programme: One year Otago programme modified for visual impairment and prescribed by physiotherapist, plus Vitamin D supplement Home safety and exercise programmes (as above) Social visits: Two one-hour visits by research staff during first 6 months of the trial to those not randomised to other groups.	Environmental hazards, risk behaviour and agreed recommendations documented at baseline Adherence evaluated at phone call (by occupational therapist) at 6 months Physiotherapist visited and telephoned participants in exercise programme during the one year Falls were measured for one year – participant given tear-off monthly postcard calendars If reported fall telephone call made to record circumstances.	• 194/198 participants allocated to home safety programme visited. 903 hazards recorded (average 4.7 per home) • 508 recommendations for change made (average 2.6 per person) • Most common recommendations: removing, replacing or modification of loose mats, repair or paint contrast strips on outside steps, outside steps handrails, improved lighting, grab rails in bathroom/toilet/shower • 169/198 (85%) had 6 month follow-up call • 152/169 (90%) reported complying partially or completely with recommendations • Average of 2.3 actions taken per person There were no differences in the number of recommendations agreed or actioned between the home safety group alone and the home safety and exercise group (recommendations p=0.446; actioned p=0.310) Falls at home associated with a hazard versus falls at home with no hazard identified were both reduced by a similar amount in participants of Home Safety Programme group compared to social visit group. This suggested that it was the advice by the occupational therapist, as well as the hazard removal which generalised to all environments enabling the person to be more environment-aware wherever they were Home safety assessment and modification in people aged over 75 with severe visual impairment significantly reduced falls when compared with social visits, where completed by an experienced occupational therapist.	Grade A – High Comments: • Relies on participant reporting all falls and recommendations • Hazards in the home assessed for those who received home safety programme only.

Source	Design and participants	Intervention	Outcomes	Results	Quality and comment
Nikolaus and Bach (2003)	Randomised controlled trial Aim: to evaluate the effect of an intervention by a multidisciplinary team to reduce falls in older people's homes Inpatients (geriatric clinic) Inclusions: • Older people • Lived at home before admission • Multiple chronic conditions or functional deterioration after convalescence, and could be discharged to home (rather than nursing home) • Lived within 15 kilometres of clinic Exclusions: terminal illness or severe cognitive decline Intervention group of 181 participants Mean age 81.2 years Male: female ratio = 50:131 Control group of 179 participants Mean age 81.9 years Male: female ratio = 44:133 Germany.	Intervention Group: Comprehensive geriatric assessment and post-discharge follow-up home visits from an interdisciplinary Home Intervention Team (HIT) HIT: three nurses, a physiotherapist, an occupational therapist, a social worker, and a secretary. One home visit during the hospital admission to evaluate the patient's home and to prescribe technical aids when necessary. To identify home hazards, a standardised home safety checklist (available in German only) was used. At least one home visit was carried out after discharge Control Group: Comprehensive geriatric assessment with recommendations followed by usual care at home. No home visit A home visit was made to all participants after 12 months.	Primary outcome: • Reduced number of falls Secondary outcomes: • Type of recommended home modifications • Compliance with recommendations • Injuries from falls.	After 1 year, 163 falls in the intervention group and 204 falls in the control group. The intervention group had 31% fewer falls than the control group (incidence rate ratio was 0.69; 95% CI [0.51,0.97]) Effectiveness of intervention greater in sub-group of participants who reported having had two or more falls during the year before recruitment to the study. The proportion of frequent fallers and the rate of falls was significantly reduced in this sub-group of the intervention group compared with the control group (21 compared to 36 participants with recurrent falls, p=0.009; incidence rate ratio was 0.63; 95% CI [0.43, 0.94]) The compliance rate varied with the type of change recommended from 83% to 33% after 12 months of follow-up A home intervention based on home visits conducted by an occupational therapist, with either a nurse or physiotherapist, to assess for environmental hazards, provide information about possible changes, facilitate any necessary home modifications, and teach the use of technical and mobility aids when necessary, was effective in a sub-group of frail older individuals with a high risk of repeated falls.	Grade A – High Comments: • Dependent on self-reporting of falls • It is not known if physical therapy in the observational period was equally distributed to both groups.

Source	Design and participants	Intervention	Outcomes	Results	Quality and comment
Nyman (2011)	Review/Overview Aim: overview of the psychosocial factors that influence older people's participation in physical activity interventions to prevent falls Multiple sources of literature.	Psychosocial factors that explain older people's participation in physical activity interventions for the prevention of falls are reviewed under the framework of the theory of planned behaviour.	Theory of planned behaviour (TPB) asserts that behaviour change is exercised through intention TPB model asserts that intention is predicted by three variables: (a) Attitude toward the behaviour (b) Subjective norm (c) Perceived behavioural control.	Implications identified from the review: Knowledge: • Opportunities for talking about and preventing non-injurious falls that may help in preventing injurious falls may be missed by health professionals • Older people's understanding of falls prevention focuses around reducing extrinsic, rather than both intrinsic and extrinsic risk factors • Older people's engagement in falls prevention interventions could be influenced by knowledge, although this was an insufficient motivator for falls prevention Attitude: • Older people were more likely to carry out falls prevention activities when they perceived that the activities would afford positive benefits and that these benefits are highly likely to occur Subjective norm: • Engagement was more likely when interventions fitted with a positive self-identity and emphasize the positive benefits of interventions, and if the older person had a high level of perceived behavioural control and a socially supportive environment Perceived behavioural control: • Participation in falls prevention interventions can be facilitated by high levels of perceived behavioural control In relation to stigma, preservation of self-identify, within the wider context of dependency is important.	Grade C – Low Comments: • Not a systematic review • Paper did not describe the search terms used to elicit papers • Much of the quoted work is by the author • One psychosocial model theory explored.

Source	Design and participants	Intervention	Outcomes	Results	Quality and comment
Nyman et al (2011)	Evaluation/Discourse analysis Aim: to explore the representations of old age in falls prevention websites and consider their potential impact on older people's uptake of advice Additionally to compare the representations against two of the Prevention of Falls Network Earth (ProFaNE) recommendations concerning fit with positive self-identify and empowerment of active self-management of health Analysis of each website and discussion to reach consensus on the emergent findings United Kingdom.	Systematic search for websites using key terms 33 websites with information on falls prevention evaluated using discourse analysis.	Ten prompts for analysis based on two recommendations from ProFaNE concerning fit with positive identity and empowerment.	Three representations of older people were identified: • The passive recipient • The rational learner • The empowered decision maker Findings demonstrated that the presentation style of online falls prevention advice is currently unlikely to be acceptable/engaging for older people, and subsequently unlikely to be effective Need identified to maximise an individual's capability and control over their own life, and as such websites must use a style that represents older people as empowered decision makers Recommendation that occupational therapists should ensure that any information produced for older people (written format or on the internet) represents them in a positive and respectful manner.	Grade C – Low Comments: • Visual data and falls prevention leaflets/pamphlets not analysed • Older people were not involved in the analysis so it cannot be claimed that the interpretation is representative of the views of older people • Only three search engines used.

Source	Design and participants	Intervention	Outcomes	Results	Quality and comment
Painter et al (2012)	Cohort study Aim: to explore • The relationship of fear of falling to depression, anxiety, activity level, and activity restriction • Whether depression or anxiety predicted fear of falling, activity level, activity restriction, or changes in activity level A convenience sampling technique using snowballing and purposive sampling was used – 7 community centres and one apartment complex Community living adults 99 participants Aged ≥ 55yrs Excluded if cognitive or developmental disability Male: female ratio = 17:82 Average age 73.71 years United Stated of America.	One 2-hour appointment A 90-minute fall prevention presentation which reviewed fall risk factors, ramifications of falls and fear of falling, home safety strategies, and community resources Sensor night light gift.	• Modified semi-structured fall questionnaire (falls history and consequences of falls in last 6 months) • Survey of Activities and Fear of Falling in the Elderly (SAFE) – assesses 11 activities both community and home based • Geriatric Depression Scale-30 • Hamilton Anxiety Scale, IVR Version.	38% reported experiencing fear of falling SAFE instrument: of the 11 activities, 88% of the participants restricted their activity level by at least one activity, and 49% indicated, compared with 5 years previously, that they were now engaging in fewer activities Activity level was negatively correlated with activity restriction, fear of falling, depression, and anxiety Anxiety predicted both fear of falling and activity level Both anxiety and depression predicted activity restriction because of fear of falling and for other reasons Overall indicated an interrelationship between the fear of falling and activity levels, fear of falling and depression and fear of falling and anxiety.	Grade C – Low Comments: • Convenience sample selection and small numbers • Heterogeneous • Self-reported data that can be subjective in nature • Questionnaire used not tested for validity or reliability • Offer of gift may have caused bias.

Source	Design and participants	Intervention	Outcomes	Results	Quality and comment
Pighills et al (2011)	Randomised controlled trial (pilot) Aim: to assess the effectiveness of an environmental falls prevention provided by qualified occupational therapists or unqualified trained assessors Recruitment via eight GP practices Inclusions: Age ≥ 70 years Community dwelling History of one or more falls over previous year Exclusions: Nursing or residential home residents and those who received falls specific occupational therapy intervention in previous year 238 participants Mean age 79 years (range 70–97) Female ratio ranged in the three arms from 62% to 71% England.	Participants randomised to one of three groups: • Occupational therapist led environmental assessment • Trained assessor led environmental assessment • Usual care control from GP and being referred for services as required Two intervention groups received: Home environment assessment using Westmead Home Safety Assessment (WeHSA) Potential falls hazards discussed, agreed recommendations. Summary of recommendations sent to participant, referrals made to other agencies for equipment and input as indicated Follow-up telephone contact after 4 weeks, and at 12 months to establish the level of adherence to recommendations and reasons for non-adherence.	Primary outcome: • Fear of falling (Falls Efficacy Scale [FES-I]) Secondary outcomes: • Falls • Quality of life (EuroQol, SF-12®) • Independence in ADL (Barthel index) Baseline measures reassessed at 3, 6 and 12 months Monthly self-completed calendars of falls Falls followed up with blinded telephone call to identify circumstances and consequences Adherence to recommendations made at four weeks and 12 months.	Follow up data for 217 participants 66% of all participants had falls Occupational therapy group had significantly less falls than unqualified (trained assessor) group at the 12 month follow-up (Incidence rate ratio was 0.54; 95% CI [0.36, 0.83]; p=0.005) There was no significant effect in the trained assessor group on falls No significant difference in fear of falling between all three groups and no effect on fear of falling The professional background of the person delivering an environmental assessment and home modification intervention influenced the effectiveness of the outcome The results indicated that occupational therapists are more effective than the non-occupational therapists in: 1. Identifying the need for modifications 2. Recommendations being adhered to 3. Smaller number of falls.	Grade A – High Comments: • Pilot study – sample size not large enough to power the study re number of falls • Minor flow diagram/text number anomaly • Limited information about the occupational therapists and trained assessors (level of experience etc).

Source	Design and participants	Intervention	Outcomes	Results	Quality and comment
Pritchard et al (2013)	Systematic review and meta-analysis Aim: to investigate the impact of falls intervention programmes on participation of older adults returning home to live, following discharge from hospital Limits were set for articles published in English, dated 1990–2012 Inclusion criteria included: • Randomised control trials • Aged ≥ 65 years • Use of an effective falls intervention and a participation measure • Post-discharge from hospital or emergency department Multiple sources of evidence.	Participation interventions were classified as such if the primary intervention used was to increase participation in life situations within the home or community settings 5 studies fulfilled the inclusion criteria and measured participation outcomes short-term (< six months post-discharge, n=488) and long-term (6–12 months post-discharge, n=571).	Participation: 'engagement in life situations' Occupation: 'engagement and participation in a recognisable everyday life endeavour' Integrating these two concepts leads to occupational participation: integrates the two concepts, involves engagement in varied activities, roles and routines that are necessary for health and wellbeing The review examined a selection of the possible occupations and assessed study outcomes against the definitions.	Interventions were classified into the following categories: • Exercise • Home modification • Psychotropic medication withdrawal • Vitamin D supplementation • Multifactorial interventions The results indicated that falls interventions provided a positive and significant improvement in the level of activities of daily living participation (p=0.042, p=0.026). However, the effect size was small at 0.20 and 0.21 Falls interventions for older adults following discharge home from hospital, increased participation in life situations to a small extent. Health professionals could include a focus on falls prevention programmes with older adults to promote participation By promoting participation in occupations that are of value to the individual and that take place in his or her everyday environments, people are more likely to be motivated to perform them long-term with positive results on participation.	Grade B – Moderate Downgraded from Grade A due to limitations: • Blinding not carried out in any of the five randomised controlled trials • Small number of studies able to be analysed impacted on the lack of generalisability of the findings • Small effect size • Varied context of the sample populations, participants at varying stages of health • Variances in the interventions carried out.

Source	Design and participants	Intervention	Outcomes	Results	Quality and comment
Rosendahl et al (2008)	Randomised controlled trial Aim: to evaluate the effectiveness of a high-intensity functional exercise programme in reducing falls in residential care facilities The study was part of Frail Older People Activity and Nutrition Study (FOPANU) 9 residential care facilities 191 participants Male: female ratio = 52:139 Aged ≥ 65 years Dependent in activities of daily living Mean ± SD score on the Mini-Mental State Examination (MMSE) was 17.8 ± 5.1 (range 10–30) Randomised to a High-Intensity Functional Exercise Program or a control activity, consisting of 29 sessions over 3 months Sweden.	Exercise Intervention: High-Intensity Functional Exercise Program (HIFE) to improve lower limb strength, balance and gait ability. The tasks were meant to be integrated into daily activities and were individually recommended Control Activity Program: Developed by occupational therapists and included activities performed in sitting e.g. watching films, reading singing and conversation The program was based on themes, e.g. the old country shop, famous people, games from the past and was expected to be interesting and stimulating for older people including those with severe cognitive impairment.	Outcome measures: • Fall rate • Proportion of participants sustaining a fall All falls were included in the study even those from epileptic seizure or acute disease Balance measured using Berg Balance Scale Analyses were based on intention to treat principle; data remained from study period start (intervention n=191, follow-up n=183) until participants died, withdrew or completed the study period The follow up period was planned to last 6 months from the end of the intervention.	During 6-month follow up (95) 52% of the 183 participants sustained one fall or more and 57 (31%) suffered more than one fall. Falls per participant ranged from 0 to 26 falls. When all participants were compared, no statistically significant differences between the groups was found for fall rate Sub-group analysis of participants who improved their balance during the intervention period indicated that the exercise group had a lower fall rate than the control group. The extent of balance improvement (of those who make an improvement in balance), did not significantly differ between exercise and control group Instead of a decline in physical function in the control group as expected, the control group activity program had an effect on physical function in the sedentary group (e.g. through the impact of social stimulation and meaningful activities, or transferring to another location in the facility) In residential care facilities a High Intensity Functional Exercise Program did not significantly reduce either fall rate or proportion of participants who sustained a fall, compared with control activity. There was however some evidence that where exercise improves balance, there may be a fall prevention effect.	Grade B – Moderate Downgraded from Grade A due to limitations: • Low statistical power. The power was slightly over 50% to show a significant reduction in falls • More participants or a longer follow up period would have been more preferable in evaluating falls • The authors state that probably not all falls were reported • Limited range of outcomes considered.

Source	Design and participants	Intervention	Outcomes	Results	Quality and comment
Schepens et al (2012)	Meta-analytic review Aims: to investigate 1. The relationships between fall-related efficacy and measures of activity and participation in community dwelling older adults 2. Whether the strength of these relationships vary depending on the type of fall-related efficacy scale and type of activity assessed Inclusions: • Conducted between 1990 and 2010 • Community living • Age ≥ 60 years • Not designated as belonging to a specific disease group Studies included non-intervention studies (e.g., cross-sectional, prospective) but excluded case reports and qualitative studies Multiple sources of evidence.	Studies had to assess fall-related efficacy using: • Falls Efficacy Scale (FES) or • Activities-specific Balance Confidence (ABC) scale Plus: • A measure of activity or participation functioning or performance Examined non-intervention studies as comparing fall-related efficacy to activity and participation.	Falls self-efficacy and balance confidence terms were pooled together for the purpose of this study and referred to as fall-related efficacy FES, ABC Scale Activity or participation functioning or performance.	20 papers on activity and 2 on participation. Activity papers showed strong positive relationship between falls-efficacy and activity An examination of 20 cross-sectional and prospective studies found a strong positive relationship between fall-related efficacy and activity (r=0.53; 95% CI [0.47, 0.58]) An insufficient number of studies examining fall-related efficacy and participation were available for analysis Highlighted importance of occupational therapists considering the impact of low fall-related efficacy as a barrier to occupational engagement for many older adults The finding of a differential effect of falls self-efficacy versus balance confidence indicated a potential need for occupational therapists to assess the two constructs separately in older adults A need was identified to consider interventions that address balance confidence and falls self-efficacy separately; this could prove beneficial and may require different strategies Study highlighted the importance for occupational therapists to focus not only on physically based outcomes but also subjective information that may influence occupational performance such as that which is gathered from measures of fall-related efficacy.	Grade B – Moderate Downgraded from Grade A due to limitations: • No assessment of quality of papers included cross sectional studies etc. • Flow chart doesn't add up correctly (1118 citations, excluded 1035 should equal 83 not 82 • Study examined the relationship of fall-related efficacy and activity at one point in time only; therefore, causality cannot be determined • Insufficient evidence to form conclusions about the relationship of fall-related efficacy to participation.

Source	Design and participants	Intervention	Outcomes	Results	Quality and comment
Stern and Jayasekara (2009)	Systematic review Aim: to determine the effectiveness of interventions designed to reduce the incidence of falls in older adult patients in acute-care hospitals compared with standard practice or no intervention Randomised controlled trials (1998 and 2008) Inclusion criteria: Aged ≥ 65 years Acute care hospitals 7 studies included in review (three based on one trial) Studies undertaken in Australia (4), UK (2) and Sweden (1).	Interventions assessed were: • Exercise • Patient Education • Vitamin D supplementation • Targeted risk factor reduction plan • 3 multifactorial intervention programmes Interventions were compared with usual care for all trials however usual care was only defined in under half of all included studies.	The outcome was the number of patient falls during hospitalisation.	In acute hospitals some evidence to suggest the following interventions may be effective in reducing the amount of falls in older people: • Multidisciplinary multifactorial intervention programme consisting of a fall risk alert card, an exercise programme, an education programme and the use of hip protectors (Haines et al 2004) • A one-on-one patient education package entailing information on risk factors and preventative strategies for falls as well as goal setting (Haines et al 2006) • A targeted fall risk factor reduction intervention that includes a fall risk factor screen, recommended interventions encompassing local advice and a summary of the evidence The authors indicate that age, morbidity, reason for hospitalisation and length of stay should be considered Some evidence to reduce number of falls was found which supported a multidisciplinary multifactorial intervention, (systematic assessment and treatment of fall risk factors and active management of post-operative complications), following surgery for femoral neck fracture.	Grade B – Moderate Downgraded from Grade A due to limitations: • Limited number of studies and lack of clarity on the search criteria • Heterogeneity across studies; data not pooled • Methodological limitations including blinding of participants to treatment groups • Not all of the intervention and control groups were treated equally • Variation in data analysis of the studies • Mix of participants across studies in terms of cognition, morbidities, age • Short length of stay (8 to 38 days), not long enough to produce significant effect.

Source	Design and participants	Intervention	Outcomes	Results	Quality and comment
Steultjens et al (2004)	Systematic review Aim: to determine if occupational therapy improves or maintains outcomes in community dwelling older people Inclusions: • Age ≥ 60 years • Living independently • Randomised controlled trials, controlled clinical trials and other designs, which may have included those with/without control • Published up to 2002 Studies evaluating multidisciplinary interventions including occupational therapy were excluded because the efficacy of occupational therapy interventions alone could not be defined definitely as causing an impact Multiple country sources of evidence assumed.	Occupational therapy regarded as: Comprehensive occupational therapy (all 5 categories below part of evaluated treatment) or 5 specific intervention categories: • Training of sensory-motor functions • Training of cognitive functions • Training of skills • Advice and instruction re use of assistive devices • Counselling of primary care giver 17 studies included, ten of which were RCTs.	Primary outcome domains: • Functional ability • Social participation • Quality of Life • Falls • Time to institutionalisation Secondary process measures: • Sensory motor functions • Cognitive functions • Depression.	The review identified evidence as follows: Strong evidence: • Efficacy of advising on assistive devices as part of home hazards assessment on functional ability Some evidence: • Efficiency of training of skills combined with home hazard assessment in decreasing incidence of falls in those at high risk of falling • Efficacy of comprehensive occupational therapy on maintaining function, quality of life and social participation of older adults Insufficient evidence was found to support the efficacy of counselling the primary care giver of older people living with dementia about maintaining their functional abilities Occupational therapy can be effective in decreasing falls for those older people at high risk of falling.	Grade B – Moderate Downgraded from Grade A due to limitations: • Included studies of different designs: RCTs, case control studies and those of other design • Several primary outcomes may bias towards positive results • Heterogeneity did not allow meta-analysis – diversity among the studies • Results are inconsistently reported and not specific enough to make any judgement about efficacy of occupational therapy interventions • No details of where original studies conducted.

Source	Design and participants	Intervention	Outcomes	Results	Quality and comment
Wijlhuizen et al (2007)	Cohort study Aim: to test the assumption that the level of outdoor physical activity mediates the relationship between fear of falling and actual outdoor falls according to the Task Difficulty Homeostasis Theory Prospective follow-up study as part of the 'Safety in your own hands study' Living independently in the community 1752 participants Age ≥ 65 years Male: female ratio = 741:1011 Recruitment via local registry office. Randomly selected 8650 and asked by mail to participate in the study 2080 (24%) agreed to participate Netherlands.	At baseline, participants were asked to complete and return a questionnaire Participants were subsequently telephoned at home once a month for 10 months and asked whether they had fallen in the previous month.	Baseline characteristics: gender, age, education, living alone, and perceived general health Asked how often afraid of falling outdoors, and, as indicator of outdoors physical activity, how often they walked outside for at least half an hour and how often they bicycled during the winter and summer During the personal telephone interview, the researchers gathered information about the nature of the fall(s) The outcome measure of the study was dichotomous: reporting at least one fall outdoors during walking or bicycling, or reporting no falls outdoors.	Data for 1752 (84%) who completed the study About 22% (n=374) of the older people reported fear of falling outside the home; 3% (n=52) had fallen outdoors during walking or bicycling in the 10-month follow-up period People with a high fear of falling were more often low to moderately active compared with people who had no such fears and were more often very active. Fear of falling was not associated with outdoor falls, but it was after taking the level of physical activity into account Found that a high fear of falling outdoors was associated with a low to moderate level of outdoor physical activity (walking, bicycling), indicating that people who perceived themselves at risk of outdoor falls adjusted their behaviour by reducing exposure Outdoor physical activity mediated the relationship between fear of falling and actual outdoor falls. This implied that the incidence of falls as an outcome in studies did not adequately represent the impact of risk factors for falls and that level of physical activity should be taken into account.	Grade C – Low Comments: • A limitation of the study was the small numbers/low (24%) proportion of participants who took part (main study required a participation commitment of about 3 years which may have discouraged the relatively older, less physically active, potential participants) • Limited to walking and bicycling • Ethics Committee did not allow the researchers to ask participants who dropped out during the follow-up for their motives.

Source	Design and participants	Intervention	Outcomes	Results	Quality and comment
Wilkins et al (2003)	Critical literature review Review question: what is the effectiveness of education and functional training programmes in improving occupational performance and quality of life for older adults? Inclusive of well older adults and/or older adults with long term conditions/ chronic illnesses Exclusions: dementia, developmental delays or mental health illness. Community-based and outpatient programmes Age ≥ 65 years. Multiple sources of evidence.	Included randomised controlled trials, cohort, single case before and after, case control and cross sectional design and case study design studies 17 articles included.	Outcomes included measurement of occupational performance, such as participation in daily activities and/or in specific areas of self-care, productivity and/or leisure outcomes, and/or environmental contexts/ conditions.	3 themes identified: a) Falls and functional decline b) Stroke c) Rheumatoid arthritis Three studies (all 1999) included on prevention of falls and implications were identified: • A medical/occupational therapy prevention approach that considers both intrinsic falls risk factors could play a significant role in reducing the number of falls and the rate of recurrent falls in older adults • In older adults with a history of falls the risk of falls, both in and outside the home could be reduced by home visits from an occupational therapist • The acceptance of home modifications by older adults might be enhanced by follow-up as well as funding • Home modifications might not be accepted and implemented by older people if there is no sense of ownership of the ideas, or opportunities for exerting control through joint decision-making and negotiation. Options and choices were important.	Grade C – Low Comments: • Critical, not systematic review • Varying quality of studies included • Limited detail of occupational therapy programmes provided in the papers reviewed • In many studies the analysis was poor or not clearly described • Most of the studies did not include long-term follow-up to enable determination of the effectiveness of the intervention over time.

Source	Design and participants	Intervention	Outcomes	Results	Quality and comment
Zijlstra et al (2007)	Systematic review Aim: to assess which interventions effectively reduce fear of falling in community-dwelling older people Inclusions: • Randomised, controlled trials with fear of falling as an outcome • Community-living older people • Mean age of 65 and older • Interventions explicitly aimed to reduce fear of falling • Interventions not explicitly aimed to reduce fear of falling Exclusions: studies targeted at people with a specific medical condition The search identified 599 abstracts, and 19 papers met the inclusion criteria Multiple sources of evidence.	Interventions explicitly aimed and interventions not explicitly aimed to reduce fear of falling were included Trials differed substantially regarding intervention characteristics and outcome measures Out of 19 trials: 8 = fall-related multifactorial interventions 3 = Tai Chi interventions 4 = exercise interventions 6 = balance interventions 1 = hip protector intervention 1 = fall risk factors 3 of the interventions explicitly aimed to reduce fear of falling.	Reduced fear of falling Most trials assessed fear of falling using the Falls Efficacy Scale (FES), Modified Falls Efficacy Scale (MFES) or an adapted version of the =ES.	In 11 trials, fear of falling was lower in the intervention group than the control group. Interventions that showed effectiveness were fall related multifactorial programs (n=5), Tai Chi interventions (n=3), exercise interventions (n=2), a hip protector intervention (n=1) The findings in trials of higher methodological quality suggested that home-based exercise and fall-related multifactorial programmes and community-based Tai Chi delivered in group format can be effective in reducing fear of falling in older people living in the community Fear of falling can be a protective response to a realistic threat and prevent people from undertaking activities with a high risk of falling and potential injury. Fear of falling can, however, result in restriction of activities that a person could safely perform which lead to unnecessary adverse consequences regarding social, mental, and physical health The experience of safely performing activities could lead to greater falls self-efficacy and a realistic view of the risk of falling.	Grade B – Moderate Downgraded from Grade A due to limitations: • Trials differed substantially regarding intervention characteristics and outcome measures • No meta-analyses conducted • Small number of trials and in seven trials, sample sizes were small, with 50 or fewer participants per group • Little attention paid to process characteristics as these are essential for understanding and improving evaluated interventions • Sub-group analyses are recommended.

ABC Scale	**Activities-specific Balance Confidence Scale**
	A 16-item self-report measure in which the person rates their balance confidence for performing activities.
	(Powell and Myers 1995)
AGS	**American Geriatrics Society**
	AGS is a not-for-profit organisation which aims to improve the health, independence and quality of life of all older people.
	http://www.americangeriatrics.org
BAOT	**British Association of Occupational Therapists**
	BAOT is the professional body for all occupational therapy staff in the United Kingdom.
	http://www.cot.co.uk/people-structure/about-baotcot
BGS	**British Geriatrics Society**
	The BGS is a professional association of health care practitioners and others with a particular interest in the medical care of older people, and in promoting better health in old age.
	http://www.bgs.org.uk
CASP	**Critical Appraisal Skills Programme**
	The Critical Appraisal Skills Programme supports the development of skills in the critical appraisal of scientific research, and provides a number of critical appraisal tools to support this activity (CASP 2013).
	http://www.casp-uk.net
CI	**Confidence Interval**
	'There is always some uncertainty in research. This is because a small group of patients is studied to predict the effects of a treatment on the wider *population*. The confidence interval is a way of expressing how certain we are about the findings from a study, using statistics. It gives a range of results that is likely to include the 'true' value for the population.
	The CI is usually stated as '95% CI', which means that the range of values has a 95 in a 100 chance of including the 'true' value. For example, a study may state that 'based on our *sample* findings, we are 95% certain that the 'true' population blood pressure is not higher than 150 and not lower than 110'. In such a case the 95% CI would be 110 to 150.
	A wide confidence interval indicates a lack of certainty about the true effect of the test or treatment - often because a small group of patients has been studied. A narrow confidence interval indicates a more precise estimate (for example, if a large number of patients have been studied).'
	Glossary: *http://www.nice.org.uk/website/glossary/glossary.jsp*

COT	**College of Occupational Therapists** COT is a wholly owned subsidiary of BAOT and operates as a registered charity. The College of Occupational Therapists sets the professional and educational standards for the occupational therapy profession and represents the profession at the national and international levels. *http://www.cot.co.uk/people-structure/about-baotcot*
COTSS-Older People	**College of Occupational Therapists Specialist Section-Older People** COTSS-Older People is a branch of the College of Occupational Therapists. It provides professional and clinical information on all aspects of occupational therapy practice related to older people. It has a responsibility to keep abreast of relevant professional, practice, policy and legislative developments and issues. Members include occupational therapy staff from both physical and mental health services for older people. *http://www.cot.co.uk/cotss-older-people/cot-ss-older-people*
DH	**Department of Health** The DH lead, shape and fund health and care in England. *https://www.gov.uk/government/organisations/department-of-health*
DHSSPSNI	**Department of Health, Social Services and Public Safety** The DHSSPSNI is a Northern Ireland Department whose mission is to improve the health and social wellbeing of the people of Northern Ireland. *http://www.dhsspsni.gov.uk*
FaB	**Falls Behavioural Scale** Evaluates behavioural factors which could potentially protect against falling. Scores range from 1 to 4, with 4 applying to the most protective behaviours. *(Clemson et al 2003)*
FES/MFES	**Falls Efficacy Scale and Modified Falls Efficacy Scale** Evaluates confidence in avoiding falls when performing basic activities of daily living. *(Hill et al 1996; Tinetti et al 1990)*
GRADE	**Grading of Recommendations Assessment, Development and Evaluation** GRADE is a systematic and explicit methodology to assist in the judgement of the quality and strength of guideline recommendations. *http://www.gradeworkinggroup.org*
HCPC	**Health and Care Professions Council** HCPC is the regulator for 16 health professions, including occupational therapists. *http://www.hcpc-uk.org*
MMSE	**Mini Mental State Examination** A series of eleven questions to test a number of mental abilities, including memory, attention and language. *(Folstein et al 1975)*

NHS	**National Health Service** The NHS refers to the publicly funded health care systems in the United Kingdom.
NICE	**National Institute for Health and Care Excellence** NICE (formerly the National Institute for Health and Clinical Excellence) provides national guidance and advice to improve health and social care. *http://www.nice.org.uk*
NOS	**National Osteoporosis Society** NOS is a United Kingdom-wide charity which is 'dedicated to improving the diagnosis, prevention and treatment of osteoporosis and fragility fractures'. *http://www.nos.org.uk*
NPSA	**National Patient Safety Agency** The NPSA leads and contributes to improved, safe patient care by informing, supporting and influencing the health sector (key functions and expertise transferred to the NHS Commissioning Board Special Health Authority in 2012). *http://www.nrls.npsa.nhs.uk*
p=values	**Probability** 'The p value is a statistical measure that indicates whether or not an effect is statistically significant. For example, if a study comparing two treatments found that one seems more effective than the other, the p value is the *probability* of obtaining these results by chance. By convention, if the p value is below 0.05 (that is, there is less than a 5% probability that the results occurred by chance) it is considered that there probably is a real difference between treatments. If the p value is 0.001 or less (less than a 1% probability that the results occurred by chance), the result is seen as highly significant. If the p value shows that there is likely to be a difference between treatments, the *confidence interval* describes how big the difference in effect might be.' *http://www.nice.org.uk/website/glossary/glossary.jsp*
ProFaNE	**Prevention of Falls Network Earth** ProFaNE was established in 2003 with the aim of increasing knowledge and capacity and thus to reduce falls amongst older people, by the implementation of evidence based intervention. *http://www.profane.eu.org*
RCT	**Randomised controlled trial** 'A study in which a number of similar people are randomly assigned to two (or more) groups to test a specific drug or treatment. One group (the experimental group) receives the treatment being tested, the other (the comparison or *control group*) receives an alternative treatment, a dummy treatment (*placebo*) or no treatment at all. The groups are followed up to see how effective the *experimental treatment* was. *Outcomes* are measured at specific times and any difference in response between the groups is assessed statistically. This method is also used to reduce *bias*.' *Glossary: http://www.nice.org.uk/website/glossary/glossary.jsp*

SF36® **SF12®**	**Health Survey** SF36® is a generic health survey that measures a person's view of their functional health and wellbeing. The 36 questions cover eight areas of physical and mental health: physical functioning; role limitations due to physical health; role limitations due to emotional problems; energy/fatigue; emotional wellbeing; social functioning; pain; and general health. The survey can be used across age, disease and treatment group. SF12® is a 12-question version of the survey.
SIGN	**Scottish Intercollegiate Guideline Network** SIGN develops evidence-based clinical practice guidelines for the National Health Service (NHS) in Scotland. *http://www.sign.ac.uk*
WeHSA	**Westmead Home Safety Assessment** The WeHSA is a 72-item checklist developed to assess the physical and environmental home hazards of people at risk of falling. Each item on the WeHSA Assessment form is first rated as being 'relevant' or 'not relevant'. For those items rated as relevant, they are then rated as a 'hazard' or 'not a hazard'. Any identified hazards are then categorised according to the listing on the assessment form. *(Clemson 1997)*

References

Evidence references

Ballinger C, Clemson L (2006) Older people's views about community falls prevention: an Australian perspective. *British Journal of Occupational Therapy, 69(6)*, 263–270.

Boltz M, Resnick B, Capezuti E, Shuluk J (2013) Activity restriction vs. self-direction: hospitalised older adults' response to fear of falling. *International Journal of Older People Nursing Jan 7.* [Epub ahead of print].

Campbell AJ, Robertson MC, La Grow SJ, Kerse NM, Sanderson GF, Jacobs RJ, Sharp DM, Hale LA (2005) Randomised controlled trial of prevention of falls in people aged ≥ 75 with severe visual impairment: the VIP trial. [Online] *British Medical Journal, 331(7520)*, 817. Available at: *http://www.bmj.com/content/331/7520/817*   Accessed on 24.11.14

Clemson L, Cumming RG, Kendig H, Swann M, Heard R, Taylor K (2004) The effectiveness of a community-based program for reducing the incidence of falls in the elderly: a randomised trial. *Journal of the American Geriatrics Society, 52(9)*, 1487–1494.

Clemson L, Mackenzie L, Ballinger C, Close JCT, Cumming RG (2008) Environmental interventions to prevent falls in community-dwelling older people: a meta-analysis of randomised trials. *Journal of Aging and Health, 20(8)*, 954–971.

Clemson L, Fiatarone Singh M, Bundy A, Cumming RG, Weissel E, Munro J, Manollaras K, Black D (2010) LiFE pilot study: a randomised trial of balance and strength training embedded in daily life activity to reduce falls in older adults. *Australian Occupational Therapy Journal, 57(1)*, 42–50.

Clemson L, Fiatarone Singh MA, Bundy A, Cumming RG, Manollaras K, O'Loughlin P, Black D (2012) Integration of balance and strength training into daily life activity to reduce rate of falls in older people (the LiFE study): randomised parallel trial. [Online] *British Medical Journal (Clinical Research Ed), 345(7870)*, 1–15. Available at: *http://dx.doi.org/10.1136/bmj.e4547*   Accessed on 24.07.14.

Costello E, Edelstein J (2008) Update on falls prevention for community-dwelling older adults: review of single and multifactorial intervention programs. *Journal of Rehabilitation Research and Development, 45(8)*, 1135–1152.

Currin ML, Comans TA, Heathcote K, Haines TP (2012) Staying safe at home. Home environmental audit recommendations and uptake in an older population at high risk of falling. *Australasian Journal on Ageing, 31(2)*, 90–95.

De Groot GC, Fagerström L (2011) Older adults' motivating factors and barriers to exercise to prevent falls. *Scandinavian Journal of Occupational Therapy, 18(2)*, 153–160.

Di Monaco M, Vallero F, De Toma E, De Lauso L, Tappero R, Cavanna A (2008) A single home visit by an occupational therapist reduces the risk of falling after hip fracture in elderly women: a quasi-randomised controlled trial. *Journal of Rehabilitation Medicine, 40(6)*, 446–450.

Di Monaco M, Vallero F, De Toma E, Castiglioni C, Gardin L, Giordano S, Tappero R (2012) Adherence to recommendations for fall prevention significantly affects the risk of falling after hip fracture: post-hoc analyses of a quasi-randomised controlled trial. *European Journal of Physical and Rehabilitation Medicine, 48(1)*, 9–15.

Gillespie LD, Robertson MC, Gillespie WJ, Sherrington C, Gates S, Clemson LM, Lamb SE (2012) Interventions for preventing falls in older people living in the community. *Cochrane Database of Systematic Reviews. Issue 9 Art. No: CD007146*. Available at: *http://dxdoi.org/10.1002/14651858.CD007146.pub3* Accessed on 29.07.14.

Gopaul K, Connelly DM (2012) Fall risk beliefs and behaviors following a fall in community-dwelling older adults: a pilot study. *Physical and Occupational Therapy in Geriatrics, 30(1)*, 53–72.

Haines TP, Bennell KL, Osborne RH, Hill KD (2004) Effectiveness of targeted falls prevention programme in subacute hospital setting: randomised controlled trial. *British Medical Journal, 328(7441)*, 676–679.

Haines TP, Hill KD, Bennell KL, Osbourne RH (2006) Patient education to prevent falls in subacute care. *Clinical Rehabilitation, 20(11)*, 970–979.

Hill A, McPhail S, Hoffmann T, Hill K, Oliver D, Beer C, Brauer S, Haines TP (2009) A randomised trial comparing digital video disc with written delivery of falls prevention education for older patients in hospital. *Journal of the American Geriatrics Society, 57(8)*, 1458–1463.

Johnston K, Barras S, Grimmer-Somers K (2010) Relationship between pre-discharge occupational therapy home assessment and prevalence of post-discharge falls. *Journal of Evaluation in Clinical Practice, 16(6)*, 1333–1339.

Kempen GI, van Haastregt JC, McKee KJ, Delbaere K, Zijlstra GA (2009) Socio-demographic, health-related and psychosocial correlates of fear of falling and avoidance of activity in community-living older persons who avoid activity due to fear of falling. *BioMed Central Public Health, 9(170)*, 1–7. Available at: *http://www.biomedcentral.com/1471-2458/9/170* Accessed on 13.08.14.

La Grow SJ, Robertson MC, Campbell AJ, Clarke GA, Kerse NM (2006) Reducing hazard related falls in people 75 years and older with significant visual impairment: how did a successful program work? *Injury Prevention, 12(5)*, 296–301.

Nikolaus T, Bach M (2003) Preventing falls in community-dwelling frail older people using a home intervention team (HIT): results from the randomised falls-HIT trial. *Journal of the American Geriatrics Society, 51(3)*, 300–305.

Nyman SR (2011) Psychosocial issues in engaging older people with physical activity interventions for the prevention of falls. *Canadian Journal on Aging, 30(1)*, 45–55.

Nyman SR, Hogarth HA, Ballinger C, Victor CR (2011) Representations of old age in falls prevention websites: implications for likely uptake of advice by older people. *British Journal of Occupational Therapy, 74(8)*, 366–374.

Painter JA, Allison L, Dhingra P, Daughtery J, Cogdill K, Trujillo LG (2012) Fear of falling and its relationship with anxiety, depression, and activity engagement among community-dwelling older adults. *American Journal of Occupational Therapy, 66(2)*, 169–176.

Pighills AC, Torgerson DJ, Sheldon TA, Drummond AE, Bland JM (2011) Environmental assessment and modification to prevent falls in older people. *Journal of The American Geriatrics Society, 59(1)*, 26–33.

Pritchard E, Brown T, Lalor A, Haines T (2013) The impact of falls prevention on participation in daily occupations of older adults following discharge: a systematic review and meta-analysis. *Disability and Rehabilitation, July 18*. [Epub ahead of print].

Rosendahl E, Gustafson Y, Nordin E, Lundin-Olsson L, Nyberg L (2008) A randomised controlled trial of fall prevention by a high-intensity functional exercise program for older people living in residential care facilities. *Aging Clinical & Experimental Research, 20(1)*, 67–75.

Schepens S, Sen A, Painter JA, Murphy SL (2011) Relationship between fall-related efficacy and activity engagement in community-dwelling older adults: a meta-analytic review. *American Journal of Occupational Therapy, 66(2)*, 137–148.

Stern C, Jayasekara R (2009) Interventions to reduce the incidence of falls in older adult patients in acute-care hospitals: a systematic review. *International Journal of Evidence-Based Healthcare, 7(4)*, 243–249.

Steultjens EMJ, Dekker J, Bouter LM, Jellema S, Bakker EB, van den Ende CHM (2004) Occupational therapy for community dwelling elderly people: a systematic review. *Age and Ageing, 33(5)*, 453–460.

Wijlhuizen GJ, de Jong R, Hopman-Rock M (2007) Older persons afraid of falling reduce physical activity to prevent outdoor falls. *Preventive Medicine, 44(3)*, 260–264.

Wilkins S, Jung B, Wishart L, Edwards M, Norton SG (2003) The effectiveness of community-based occupational therapy education and functional training programs for older adults: a critical literature review. *Canadian Journal of Occupational Therapy, 70(4)*, 214–225.

Zijlstra G, van Haastregt J, van Rossum E, van Eijk J, Yardley L, Kempen G (2007) Interventions to reduce fear of falling in community-living older people: a systematic review. *Journal of the American Geriatrics Society, 55(4)*, 603–615.

Supporting information references

Age UK, National Osteoporosis Society (2012) *Report to the Minister of State for Care Services. Breaking through: building better falls and fracture services in England.* London: Age UK. Available at: *http://www.nos.org.uk/document.doc?id=987*
Accessed on 19.03.14.

Age UK (2014) *Later life in the United Kingdom*. London: Age UK. Available at: *http://www.ageuk.org.uk/Documents/EN-GB/Factsheets/Later_Life_UK_factsheet.pdf?dtrk=true*
Accessed on 13.08.14.

Alzheimer's Society (2009) *Counting the cost: caring for people with dementia on hospital wards*. London: Alzheimer's Society. Available at: *http://www.alzheimers.org.uk/site/scripts/documents_info.php?documentID=1199*
Accessed on 19.03.14.

American Geriatrics Society, British Geriatrics Society, American Academy of Orthopaedic Surgeons Panel on Falls Prevention (2001) Guideline for the prevention of falls in older persons. *Journal of the American Geriatrics Society, 49(5)*, 664–672.

American Geriatrics Society, British Geriatrics Society [ca. 2010] *AGS/BGS Clinical Practice Guideline: prevention of falls in older persons*. New York: American Geriatrics Society. Available at: *http://www.medcats.com/FALLS/frameset.htm*
Accessed on 20.03.14.

Aragon A, Kings J (2010) *Occupational therapy for people with Parkinson's*. London: COT. Available at: *http://www.cot.co.uk/sites/default/files/publications/public/OT-People-Parkinsons.pdf*
Accessed on 07.04.14.

Australian Commission on Safety and Quality in Healthcare (2009a) *Guidebook for preventing falls and harm from falls in older people: Australian community care. A short version of Preventing falls and harm from falls in older people: best practice guidelines for Australian community care*. Sydney: Commonwealth of Australia. Available at: *http://www.safetyandquality.gov.au/wp-content/uploads/2012/01/30455-COMM-Guidebook1.pdf*
Accessed on 21.03.14.

Australian Commission on Safety and Quality in Healthcare (2009b) *Guidebook for preventing falls and harm from falls in older people: Australian hospitals. A short version of Preventing falls and harm from falls in older people: best practice guidelines for Australian hospitals*. Sydney: Commonwealth of Australia. Available at: *http://www.safetyandquality.gov.au/wp-content/uploads/2012/01/30459-HOSP-Guidebook1.pdf*
Accessed on 21.03.14.

Australian Commission on Safety and Quality in Healthcare (2009c) *Guidebook for preventing falls and harm from falls in older people: Australian residential aged care facilities. A short version of Preventing falls and harm from falls in older people: best practice guidelines for Australian residential aged care facilities*. Sydney: Commonwealth of Australia. Available at: *http://www.safetyandquality.gov.au/wp-content/uploads/2012/01/30454-RACF-Guidebook1.pdf*
Accessed on 21.03.14.

Baker SP, Harvey AH (1985) Fall injuries in the elderly. *Clinical Geriatric Medicine, 1(3)*, 501–512.

Ballinger C, Brooks C (2013) *An overview of best practice for falls prevention from an occupational therapy perspective*. London: Health Foundation. Available at: *http://patientsafety.health.org.uk/sites/default/files/resources/an_overview_of_best_practice_for_falls_prevention_from_an_occupational_therapy_perspective_0.pdf*
Accessed on 30.06.14.

Banerjee J, Conroy S (2012) *Quality care for older people with urgent & emergency care needs*. London: British Geriatrics Society. Available at: *http://www.bgs.org.uk/campaigns/silverb/silver_book_complete.pdf*
Accessed on 21.03.14.

[British Orthopaedic Association] (2007) *The care of patients with fragility fracture.* London: BOA. Available at: *http://www.nhfd.co.uk/20/hipfractureR.nsf/luMenu Definitions/FCEF9FCB98A1B8EB802579C900553996/$file/Blue_Book.pdf?OpenElement* Accessed on 14.08.14.

Bunn F, Dickinson A, Simpson C, Narayanan V, Humphrey D, Griffiths C, Martin W, Victor C (2014) Preventing falls among older people with mental health problems: a systematic review. [Online] *BioMed Central Nursing. Available at: http://www.biomedcentral.com/ content/pdf/1472-6955-13-4.pdf* Accessed on 11.04.14.

Chase CA, Mann K, Wasek S, Arbesman M (2012) Systematic review of the effect of home modification and fall prevention programs on falls and the performance of community-dwelling older adults. *American Journal of Occupational Therapy, 66(3),* 272–276.

Clemson L (1997) *Home fall hazards: A guide to identifying fall hazards in the homes of elderly people and an accompaniment to the assessment tool, the Westmead Home Safety Assessment.* West Brunswick, Victoria, Australia: Coordinates Publication.

Clemson L, Cusick A, Fozzard C (1999) Managing risk and exerting control: determining follow through with falls prevention. *Disability and Rehabilitation, 21,* 1321–1326.

Clemson L, Cumming RG, Heard R (2003) The development of an assessment to evaluate behavioural factors associated with falling. *American Journal of Occupational Therapy, 57(4),* 380–388.

Close J, Ellis M, Hooper R, Glucksman E, Jackson S, Swift C (1999) Prevention of falls in the elderly trial (PROFET): a randomised control trial. *Lancet, 353(9147),* 93–97.

College of Occupational Therapists (2006) *Falls management.* London: COT.

College of Occupational Therapists (2007) *Building the evidence for occupational therapy: priorities for research.* London: COT. Available at: *http://www.cot.co.uk/ publication/books-z-listing/building-evidence-occupational-therapy-priorities-research* Accessed on 30.04.14.

College of Occupational Therapists (2010) *Code of ethics and professional conduct.* London: COT. Available at: *http://www.cot.co.uk/sites/default/files/publications/public/ Code-of-Ethics2010.pdf* Accessed on 30.04.14.

College of Occupational Therapists (2011a) *Practice guidelines development manual.* 2nd ed. London: COT. Available at: *http://www.cot.co.uk/sites/default/files/publications/ public/PGD-Manual-2014.pdf* Accessed on 30.04.14.

College of Occupational Therapists (2011b) *Professional standards for occupational therapy practice.* London: COT. Available at: *http://www.cot.co.uk/standards-ethics/ professional-standards-occupational-therapy-practice* Accessed on 30.04.14.

College of Occupational Therapists (2011c) *Occupational therapy with people who have had lower limb amputations: evidence-based guidelines.* London: COT. Available at: *http://www.cot.co.uk/sites/default/files/publications/public/Lower-Limb-Guidelines[1].pdf* Accessed on 30.04.14.

College of Occupational Therapists (2012) *Occupational therapy for adults undergoing total hip replacement: practice guideline.* London: COT. Available at: *http://www.cot. co.uk/sites/default/files/publications/public/P171-Total-Hip-replacement.pdf*
Accessed on 24.03.14.

College of Occupational Therapists (2013a) *Occupational therapists' use of standardised outcome measures.* London: COT. Available at: *http://www.cot.co.uk/sites/default/files/ position_statements/public/COT%20Position%20Statement%20-%20measuring%20 outcomes.pdf*
Accessed on 20.03.14.

College of Occupational Therapists (2013b) *Living well through activity in care home: the toolkit.* London: COT. Available at: *http://www.cot.co.uk/living-well-care-homes*
Accessed on 08.04.14.

College of Occupational Therapists (2014) *OT Subset: assessment tools.* London: COT. Available at: *http://www.cot.co.uk/ehealth-information-management/ot-subset-assessment-tools*
Accessed on 17.04.14.

College of Optometrists (2014) *Focus on falls.* London: College of Optometrists. Available at: *http://www.college-optometrists.org/en/EyesAndTheNHS/focus-on-falls.cfm*
Accessed on 11.04.14.

Connell BR, Wolf SL (1997) Environmental and behavioural circumstances associate with falls at home among healthy elderly individuals. *Archives of Physical Medical Rehabilitation, 78(2),* 179–186.

Cox CR, Clemson L, Stancliffe RJ, Durvasula S, Sherrington C (2010) Incidence of and risk factors for falls among adults with an intellectual disability. *Journal of Intellectual Disability Research, 54(12),* 1045–1057.

Critical Appraisal Skills Programme (2013) *CASP checklists.* Oxford: CASP. Available at: *http://www.casp-uk.net/*
Accessed on 20.03.14.

Cummings RB, Thomas M, Szonyi G, Salkeld G, O'Neill E, Westbury C, Frampton G (1999) Home visits by an occupational therapist for assessment and modification of environmental hazards: a randomised trial of falls prevention. *Journal of the American Geriatrics Society, 47(12),* 1397–1402.

Cummings RB, Salkeld G, Thomas M, Szonyi G (2000) Prospective study of the impact of fear of falling in activities of daily living, SF-36 scores and nursing home admission. *Journal of Gerontology, 55(5),* 299–305.

Czernuszenko A, Członkowska A (2009) Risk factors for falls in stroke patients during inpatient rehabilitation. *Clinical Rehabilitation, 23(2),* 176–188.

Department of Health (2001) *National Service Framework for Older People.* London: DH. Available at: *https://www.gov.uk/government/uploads/system/uploads/attachment_data/ file/198033/National_Service_Framework_for_Older_People.pdf*   Accessed on 19.03.14.

Department of Health (2009) *Falls and fractures: effective interventions in health and social care.* London: DH. Available at: *http://www.slips-online.co.uk/resources/ Fallsandfractures-effectiveinterventionsinhealthandsocialcare.pdf* Accessed on 19.03.14.

Department of Health (2010) *Prevention package for older people resources.* London: DH. Available at: *http://www.webarchive.nationalarchives.gov.uk/+/www.dh.gov.uk/en/ Publicationsandstatistics/Publications/DH_103146*   Accessed on 24.06.14.

Department of Health (2013a) *Improving quality of life for people with long term conditions.* London: DH. Available at: *https://www.gov.uk/government/policies/ improving-quality-of-life-for-people-with-long-term-conditions*   Accessed on 09.04.14.

Department of Health (2013b) *Integration pioneers leading the way for health and care reform.* London: DH. Available at: *https://www.gov.uk/government/news/integration- pioneers-leading-the-way-for-health-and-care-reform--2*   Accessed on 01.07.14.

Department of Health (2014) *Enabling integrated care in the NHS.* London: DH. Available at: *https://www.gov.uk/enabling-integrated-care-in-the-nhs*
                                                                  Accessed on 30.06.14.

Department of Health, Public Health England (2014) *A framework for personalised care and population health for nurse, midwives, health visitors and allied health professionals. Caring for populations across the life course.* London: DH and Public Health England. Available at: *https://www.gov.uk/government/uploads/system/uploads/ attachment_data/file/326984/PHP_Framework_Version_1.pdf*   Accessed on 08.07.14.

Department of Health, Social Services and Public Safety (2012) *Living with long term conditions: a policy framework.* Belfast: DHSSPSNI. Available at: *http://www.dhsspsni. gov.uk/living-longterm-conditions.pdf*   Accessed on 23.06.14.

Department of Health, Social Services and Public Safety (2013) *Service Framework for Older People.* Belfast: DHSSPSNI. Available at: *http://www.dhsspsni.gov.uk/service_ framework_for_older_people-2.pdf*   Accessed on 19.03.14.

Department of Health, Social Services and Public Safety (2014) *Transforming your care.* Belfast: DHSSPSNI. Available at: *http://www.transformingyourcare.hscni.net/*
                                                                  Accessed on 30.06.14.

De Silva D (2014) *Helping measure person-centred care.* London: Health Foundation. Available at: *http://www.health.org.uk/publications/helping-measure-person-centred- care*   Accessed on 19.03.14.

Dyer CAE, Taylor GJ, Reed M, Dyer CA, Robertson DR, Harrington R (2004) Falls prevention in residential care homes: a randomised controlled trial. *Age and Ageing, 33(6),* 596–602.

Finlayson M, Peterson EW, Cho C (2009) Pilot study of a fall risk management program for middle aged and older adults with MS. *Neurorehabilitation, 25(2),* 107–115.

Folstein MF, Folstein SE, McHugh PR (1975) Mini Mental State: a practical method for grading the cognitive state of patients for the clinician. *Journal of Pschiatric Research, 12(3),* 189–198.

Gitlin LN, Hauck WW, Winter L, Dennis MP, Schulz R (2006) Effect of an in-home occupational and physical therapy intervention on reducing mortality in functionally vulnerable older people: preliminary findings. *Journal of the American Geriatrics Society, 54(6),* 950–955.

GRADE Working Group (2004) Grading quality of evidence and strength of recommendations. *British Medical Journal, 328(7454)*, 1490–1494.

Gryfe CI, Amies A, Ashley MJ (1977) A longitudinal study of falls in an elderly population: incidence and morbidity. *Age and Ageing, 6(4)*, 201–210

Guyatt GH, Oxman AD, Kunz R, Falck-Ytter Y, Vist GE, Liberati A, Schünemann HJ, GRADE Working Group (2008) Rating quality of evidence and strength of recommendations: going from evidence to recommendations. *British Medical Journal, 336(7652)*, 1049–1051.

Hawley-Hague H, Boulton E, Hall A, Pfeiffer K, Todd C (2014) Older adults' perceptions of technologies aimed at falls prevention, detection or monitoring: a systematic review. *International Journal of Medical Informatics, April 1*. [Epub ahead of print].
Accessed on 30.04.14.

Health and Care Professions Council (2013) *Standards of proficiency: occupational therapists.* London: HCPC. Available at: *http://www.hcpc-uk.org/assets/ documents/10000512Standards_of_Proficiency_Occupational_Therapists.pdf*
Accessed on 20.03.14.

Health and Care Professions Council (2012) *Standards of conduct, performance and ethics.* London: HCPC. Available at: *http://www.hcpc-uk.org/assets/documents/10003B6ES tandardsofconduct,performanceandethics.pdf* Accessed on 20.03.14.

Henderson C, Beecham J, Knapp M (2013) The costs of telecare and telehealth In: L Curtis, ed. *Unit costs of health and social care 2013*. Canterbury: Personal Social Services Research Unit. 26–31. Available at: *http://www.pssru.ac.uk/project-pages/unit-costs/2013/*
Accessed on 20.03.14.

Hill KD, Schwarz JA, Kalogeropoulos AJ, Gibson SJ (1996). Fear of falling revisited. *Archives of Physical Medicine and Rehabilitation*, 77(10), 1025–1029.

Hindle L (2014) AHPs an integral part of the public health workforce. London: Public Health England. Available at: *http://www.cot.co.uk/sites/default/files/general/public/ Linda-Hindle-S1.pptx* Accessed on 30.06.14.

Horton K (2008) Falls in older people: the place of telemonitoring in rehabilitation. *Journal of Rehabilitation Research and Development, 45(8)*, 1183–1194.

Irvine L, Conroy SP, Sach T, Gladman JR, Harwood RH, Kendrick D, Coupland C, Drummond A, Barton G, Masud T (2010) Cost-effectiveness of a day hospital falls prevention programme for screened community-dwelling older people at high risk of falls. *Age and Ageing, 39(6)*, 710–716.

Law M, Cooper B, Strong S, Steward D, Rigby P, Letts L (1996) The person-environment occupation model: a transactive approach to occupational performance. *Canadian Journal of Occupational Therapy, 63(1)*, 9–22.

Lee JE, Stokic DS (2008) Risk factors for falls during inpatient rehabilitation. *American Journal of Physical Medicine & Rehabilitation, 87(5)*, 341–350.

Legood R, Scuffham P, Cryer C (2002) Are we blind to injuries in the visually impaired? A review of the literature. *Injury Prevention, 8(2)*, 155–160. Available at: *http://injuryprevention.bmj.com/content/8/2/155.full.pdf+html*   Accessed on 19.03.14.

Mackenzie L, Clemson L (2014) Can chronic disease management plans including occupational therapy and physiotherapy services contribute to reducing falls risk in older people? *Australian Family Physician, 43(4)*, 211–215. Available at: *http://www.racgp.org.au/download/Documents/AFP/2014/April/201404Mackenzie.pdf*
Accessed on 28.04.14.

Marmot M (2010) *Fair society, healthy lives: the Marmot review*. [London]: Marmot Review. Available at: *http://www.ucl.ac.uk/whitehallII/pdf/FairSocietyHealthyLives.pdf*
Accessed on 19.03.14.

Martin M (2013) *Falls in older people with sight loss: a review of emerging research and key action points*. (*Research Discussion Paper 12*). London: Thomas Pocklington Trust. Available at: *http://www.pocklington-trust.org.uk/Resources/Thomas%20Pocklington/Documents/PDF/Research%20Publications/RDP%2012_final.pdf*   Accessed on 19.03.14.

Masud T, Morris RO (2001) Epidemiology of falls. *Age and Ageing, 30(S4)*, 3–7.

Morris JC, Rubin EH, Morris EJ, Mandel SA (1987) Senile dementia of the Alzheimer's type: an important risk factor for serious falls. *Journal of Gerontology, 42(4)*, 12–17.

Murray G, Cameron I, Cumming R (2007) The consequences of falls in acute and subacute hospitals in Australia that cause proximal femoral fractures. *Journal of the American Geriatrics Society, 55(4)*, 577–582.

National Institute for Health and Clinical Excellence (2004) *The assessment and prevention of falls in older people*. (Clinical Guideline CG21). London: NICE.

National Institute for Health and Clinical Excellence (2008) *Occupational therapy and physical activity interventions to promote the mental wellbeing of older people in primary care and residential care*. (Public Health Guidance 16). London: NICE. Available at: *http://www.nice.org.uk/guidance/ph16/resources/guidance-occupational-therapy-and-physical-activity-interventions-to-promote-the-mental-wellbeing-of-older-people-in-primary-care-and-residential-care-pdf*   Accessed on 11.07.14.

National Institute for Health and Clinical Excellence (2011) *Hip fracture: the management of hip fracture in adults*. (Clinical Guideline 124). London: NICE. Available at: *http://www.nice.org.uk/nicemedia/live/13489/54919/54919.pdf*   Accessed on 21.03.14.

National Institute for Health and Clinical Excellence (2012a) *Quality standard for hip fracture*. (Quality Standard 16). London: NICE. Available at: *http://publications.nice.org.uk/quality-standard-for-hip-fracture-qs16*   Accessed on 24.03.14.

National Institute for Health and Care Excellence (2012b) *Osteoporosis: assessing the risk of fragility fracture*. (Clinical Guideline 146). London: NICE. Available at: *http://www.nice.org.uk/nicemedia/live/13857/60399/60399.pdf*   Accessed on 21.03.14.

National Institute for Health and Care Excellence (2013a) *Action needed to reduce hospital falls: a 'one size fits all' approach will not work, warns NICE*. London: NICE. Available at: *https://www.nice.org.uk/News/Article/older-patients-at-high-risk-of-hospital-falls*   Accessed on 19.03.14.

National Institute for Health and Care Excellence (2013b) *Falls: assessment and prevention of falls in older people. Costing statement.* London: NICE. Available at: *http://www.nice.org.uk/guidance/cg161/resources/cg161-falls-costing-statement2*
Accessed on 30.06.14.

National Institute for Health and Care Excellence (2013c) *Falls: the assessment and prevention of falls in older people.* (Clinical Guideline CG161). London: NICE. Available at: *http://www.nice.org.uk/nicemedia/live/14181/64166/64166.pdf* Accessed on 19.03.14.

National Institute for Health and Care Excellence (2014) *Falls in older people NICE Pathway.* London: NICE. Available at: *http://pathways.nice.org.uk/pathways/falls-in-older-people*
Accessed on 24.06.14.

National Institute for Health and Care Excellence (In press) *Quality standard for falls.* London: NICE.

National Patient Safety Agency (2007) *Slips, trips and falls in hospital.* London: NPSA. Available at: *http://www.nrls.npsa.nhs.uk/resources/collections/pso-reports/?entryid45=59821*
Accessed on 19.03.14.

NHS Centre for Reviews and Dissemination (1996) *Preventing falls and subsequent injury in older people. Effective Health Care, 2(4)*, 1–16. Available at: *https://www.york.ac.uk/inst/crd/EHC/ehc24.pdf*
Accessed on 12.08.14.

NHS Confederation (2012) *Falls prevention: new approaches to integrated falls prevention services. (Issue 234).* London: NHS Confederation. Available at: *http://www.nhsconfed.org/Publications/Documents/Falls_prevention_briefing_final_for_website_30_April.pdf*
Accessed on 19.03.14.

NHS Quality Improvement Scotland (2010) *Up and about pathways for the prevention and management of falls and fragility fractures.* Edinburgh: Healthcare Improvement Scotland. Available at: *http://www.healthcareimprovementscotland.org/default.aspx?page=13131*
Accessed on 19.03.14.

Office for National Statistics (2013) *National Population Projections 2012-based Statistical Bulletin.* Newport: ONS. Available at: *http://www.ons.gov.uk/ons/dcp171778_334975.pdf*
Accessed on 14.08.14.

Parry SW, Finch T, Deary V (2013) How should we manage fear of falling in older adults living in the community? [Online] *British Medical Journal, 346 (1)*, f2933. Available at: *http://dx.doi.org/10.1136/bmj.f2933*
Accessed on 13.08.14.

Patient Safety First (2009) *The 'how to' guide for reducing harm from falls.* London: Patient Safety First. Available at: *http://www.patientsafetyfirst.nhs.uk/ashx/Asset.ashx?path=/Intervention-support/FALLSHow-to%20Guide%20v4.pdf*
Accessed on 19.03.14.

Powell LE, Myers AM (1985) The Activities-specific Balance Confidence (ABC) Scale. [Online] *Journal of Gerontology, 50(1)*, M28–M34. Available at: http://biomedgerontology.oxfordjournals.org/content/50A/1/M28.abstract
Accessed on 12.08.14

Richardson WS, Wilson MC, Nishikawa J, Hayward RS (1995) The well-built clinical question: a key to evidence-based decisions. *ACP J Club, 123(3)*,A12–a13.

Royal College of Physicians (2012) *Report of the 2011 inpatient falls pilot audit*. London: RCP. Available at: *https://www.rcplondon.ac.uk/sites/default/files/inpatient-falls-final-report.pdf*　　　　Accessed on 30.06.14.

Royal College of Physicians (2010) *Falling standards, broken promises: report of the national audit of falls and bone health in older people 2010*. London: RCP. Available at: *https://www.rcplondon.ac.uk/sites/default/files/national_report_0.pdf*
　　　　Accessed on 19.03.14.

Saverino A, Moriarty A, Playford D (2013) The risk of falling in young adults with neurological conditions: a systematic review. *Disability and Rehabilitation, Oct 7*. [Epub ahead of print].

Scotland. Scottish Government (2012) *AHPs as agents of change in health and social care: the National Delivery Plan for the allied health professions in Scotland, 2012–2015*. Edinburgh: Scottish Government. Available at: *http://www.scotland.gov.uk/Resource/0039/00395491.pdf*　　　　Accessed on 19.03.14.

Scotland. Scottish Government (2013) *Long term conditions*. Edinburgh: Scottish Government. Available at: *http://www.scotland.gov.uk/Topics/Health/Services/Long-Term-Conditions*　　　　Accessed on 09.04.14.

Scotland. Scottish Government (2014) *Integration of health and social care*. Edinburgh: Scottish Government. Available at: *http://www.scotland.gov.uk/Topics/Health/Policy/Adult-Health-SocialCare-Integration*　　　　Accessed on 30.06.14.

Scottish Intercollegiate Guidelines Network (2003) *Management of osteoporosis*. (National Clinical Guideline Number 71). Edinburgh: SIGN. Available at: *http://sign.ac.uk/pdf/sign71.pdf*　　　　Accessed on 21.03.14.

Scottish Intercollegiate Guidelines Network (2009) *Management of hip fracture in older people*. (National Clinical Guideline Number 111). Edinburgh: SIGN. Available at: *http://www.sign.ac.uk/pdf/sign111.pdf*　　　　Accessed on 21.03.14.

Scuffham P, Chaplin S, Legood R (2003) Incidence and costs of unintentional falls in older people in the UK. *Journal of Epidemiological Community Health, 57(9)*, 740–747.

Shaw FE, Bond J, Richardson DA, Dawson P, Steen IN, McKeith IG, Kenny RA (2003) Multifactorial intervention after a fall in older people with cognitive impairment and dementia presenting to the accident and emergency department: randomised controlled trial. *British Medical Journal, 326(7380)*, 73–75.

Social Care and Social Work Improvement Scotland, NHS Scotland (2011). *Managing falls and fractures in care homes for older people. Good practice self assessment resource*. Edinburgh: SCSWIS. Available at: *http://www.careinspectorate.com/index.php?option=com_docman&task=cat_view&gid=329&Itemid=720*　　　　Accessed on 19.03.14.

Social Care Institute for Excellence, College of Occupational Therapists (2011) *Reablement: a key role for occupational therapists.* (At a glance 46) London: SCIE. Available at: *http://www.scie.org.uk/publications/ataglance/ataglance46.asp*
Accessed on 30.06.14.

Stalenhoef PA, Diederiks JPM, Knottnerus JA, Kester ADM, Crebolder HFJM (2002) A risk model for the prediction of recurrent falls in community-dwelling elderly: a prospective cohort study. *Journal of Clinical Epidemiology, 55(11),* 1088–1094.

Steventon A, Bardsley M, Billings J, Dixon J, Doll H, Beynon M, Hirani S, Cartwright M, Rixon L, Knapp M, Henderson C, Rogers A, Hendy J, Fitzpatrick R, Newman S (2013) Effect of telecare on use of health and social care services: findings from the Whole Systems Demonstrator cluster randomised trial. *Age and Ageing, 42(4),* 501–508. Available at: *http://ageing.oxfordjournals.org/content/42/4/501.full.pdf+html*
Accessed on 20.03.14.

Stewart LS, McKinstry B (2012) Fear of falling and the use of telecare by older people. *British Journal of Occupational Therapy, 75(7),* 304–312.

Tian Y, Thompson J, Buck D, Sonola L (2013) *Exploring the system-wide cost of falls in older people in Torbay.* London: King's Fund. Available at: *http://www.kingsfund.org.uk/ sites/files/kf/field/field_publication_file/exploring-system-wide-costs-of-falls-in-torbay-kingsfund-aug13.pdf*
Accessed on 27.06.14.

Tinetti ME (1987) Factors associated with serious injury during falls by ambulatory nursing home patients. *Journal of the American Geriatrics Society, 35(7),* 644–648.

Tinetti ME, Speechley M, Ginter SF (1998) Risk factors for falls among elderly persons living in the community. *New England Journal of Medicine, 319(26),* 1701–1707.

Tinetti ME, Richman D. Powell L (1990) Falls efficacy as a measure of falling. *Journal of Gerontology, 45(6),* 239–243.

Tolley L, Atwal A (2003) Determining the effectiveness of a falls prevention programme to enhance quality of life: an occupational therapy perspective. *British Journal of Occupational Therapy, 66(6),* 269–276.

Van Dijk PTM, Meulenberg OGRM, Van De Sande HJ, Habbema JDK (1993) Falls in dementia patients. *Gerontologist, 33(2),* 200–204.

Voss T, Flaxman AD, Naghavi M, Lozano R, Michaud C, Ezzati M et al (2012) Years lived with disability (YLDs) for 1160 sequelae of 289 diseases and injuries 1990—2010: a systematic analysis for the Global Burden of Disease Study 2010. *Lancet, 380 (9859),* 2163–2196.

Wales Audit Office (2014) *The management of chronic conditions in Wales: an update.* Cardiff: Wales Audit Office. Available at: *http://www.wao.gov.uk/system/files/ publications/The%20Management%20of%20Chronic%20Conditions%20in%20 Wales%20-%20An%20Update.pdf*
Accessed on 23.06.14.

Wales. Welsh Assembly Government (2006) *THe National Service Framework for Older People in Wales.* Cardiff: Welsh Assembly Government. Available at: *http://www.wales. nhs.uk/sites3/documents/439/NSFforOlderPeopleInWalesEnglish.pdf*
Accessed on 19.03.14.

Wales. Welsh Government (2014) *A framework for delivering integrated health and social care for older people with complex needs.* Cardiff: Welsh Government. Available at: *http://wales.gov.uk/topics/health/publications/socialcare/strategies/integration/?lang=en*   Accessed on 30.06.14.

Wesson J, Clemson L, Brodaty H, Lord S, Taylor M, Gitlin L, Close J (2013) A feasibility study and pilot randomised trial of a tailored prevention program to reduce falls in older people with mild dementia. *BioMed Central Geriatrics, 13(1),* 89.

Wijlhuizen GJ, Chorus AM, Hopman-Rock M (2008) The 24-h distribution of falls and person-hours of physical activity in the home are strongly associated among community-dwelling older persons. *Preventive Medicine, 46(6),* 605–608.

Wijlhuizen GJ, Chorus AM, Hopman-Rock M (2010) The FARE: a new way to express Falls Risk among older persons including physical activity as a measure of exposure. *Preventive Medicine, 50(3),* 143–147.

Willgoss TA (2010) Falls in people with learning disabilities: what are the risk factors and prevention strategies? *Nursing Times, 106(46),* 10–12.

Winter H, Watt K, Peel NM (2013) Falls prevention interventions for community-dwelling older persons with cognitive impairment: a systematic review. *International Psychogeriatrics, 25(2),* 215–227.

Yardley L. Donovan-Hall M, Francis K, Todd C (2006) Older people's views of advice about falls prevention: a qualitative study. *Health Education Research Theory and Practice, 21(4),* 508–517.

Yardley L, Beyer N, Hauer K, McKee K, Ballinger C, Todd C (2007) Recommendations for promoting the engagement of older people in activities to prevent falls. *Quality & Safety in Health Care, 16(3),* 230–234.

Yardley L, Kirby S, Ben-Shlomo Y, Gilbert R, Whitehead S, Todd C (2008) How likely are older people to take up different falls prevention activities? *Preventive Medicine, 47(5),* 554–558.